T0246077

Take Charge of Your Own Ageing

By 2046, 36% of Hong Kongers will be 'older adults'. *Take Charge of Your Own Ageing* is a timely publication to remind our society about the significance of co-creating a city that is environmentally and socially friendly towards the physical, mental and social well-being of an ageing population with a 100-year lifespan. This book is a must-read for policymakers, businessmen, NGOs, older adults and caregivers. Collaborative and intersectoral efforts are needed to foster age-friendly policies, measures and places, empowering older adults to take charge of their own lives instead of being passive care recipients.

—Professor Ng Mee Kam
Director, Urban Studies Programme, CUHK

Even in her seventies, Professor Jean Woo has kept the fire in her heart burning. With her unwavering commitment to health, she herself is a demonstration of living a life to the fullest against a ticking clock. Not only is she outspoken, but she also takes seriously her commitment to improving the health of Hong Kong people through community services, gerontechnology, and countless studies on well-being.

This book records what Prof. Woo, as an authority of on gerontology, has observed in the hospitals and communities in Hong Kong over the past half century. She is frank enough to point out the various problems behind the façade of Hong Kong people's longevity: How can the health indicators of the elderly be the same as those of the general population? Apart from the general differences in health problems and treatments between men and women, the elderly also suffer from deleterious effects of loneliness and social isolation after the pandemic as the outcome of health inequalities.

— Chan Hiu Lui
Chief Editor of Big Silver

Over the past two to three decades, the WHO has endeavoured to promote universal health and develop primary healthcare, emphasising that collective efforts from various sectors of society are necessary to achieve good health for all, and maintain the quality of life in old age by improving areas ranging from urban design, public services, private market operations, education, employment, housing, food safety, to social inclusion, community participation, and poverty eradication. In other words, we need to plan for a 'healthy city'. Both Prof. Woo and I have happened to promote interdisciplinary and trans-sectoral collaboration within communities, to encourage everyone to take their awareness of health to the next level— taking appropriate health actions with improved health literacy.

I hope for a complete change in Hong Kong society, whether it is a change in our vision of life or our social culture and socio-economic operations that prompt us to think only the healthcare system is responsible for handling wellbeing issues. Just as Prof. Woo said we cannot simply 'relying on doctors, investigations and drugs, accompanied by unrealistic expectations that bad health outcomes can be avoided if you do what the doctors tell you'. After all, why do we strive to maintain good health? Isn't it because there is nothing more important than living well and dying well?

—**Dr Fan Ning**
Founder of Health In Action & Chairman of Forget Thee Not

TAKE CHARGE OF
YOUR OWN AGEING
GROWING OLD IN HONG KONG

Jean Woo

The Chinese University of Hong Kong Press

Take Charge of Your Own Ageing: Growing Old in Hong Kong
By Jean Woo

© The Chinese University of Hong Kong 2024

ISBN: 978-988-237-313-6

The Chinese University of Hong Kong Press
The Chinese University of Hong Kong
Sha Tin, N.T., Hong Kong
Fax: +852 2603 7355
Email: cup@cuhk.edu.hk
Website: cup.cuhk.edu.hk

Printed in Hong Kong

CONTENTS

PREFACE

As I write this, I am in my seventh decade, having worked as a teacher, researcher and doctor in Hong Kong since 1977. My family emigrated to London in 1960, where I attended secondary school and university, subsequently working in various specialties in London hospitals. My personal experience of ageing covers my experience with my family in the UK, as well as my husband's family in Hong Kong. My work experience covers a period working part time in the private sector in general practice, and then for many years in the public hospital sector, setting up the geriatric service in the New Territories East Cluster in 1985 after joining the newly established Department of Medicine of The Chinese University of Hong Kong. At that time, academics led the service development, teaching and research in hospitals run by the Hospital Authority. I remember the profile of patients in the medical wards were very different: there were very few people aged 60 and above. A patient with a diagnosis of dementia created so much excitement that the newly established specialty of Psychogeriatrics immediately took the patient over to their wards. Practically everyone could walk to the toilet and eat by themselves. By the time I retired from regular hospital work approximately 30 years later, the majority of patients in medical wards were aged 80 to 100 and could not or were not allowed to get to the toilet. Use of restraints was common in the name of safety, as were incontinence pads. During wintertime, most of the patients admitted from Residential Care Homes for the Elderly (RCHEs) were bedridden, and sometimes up to one third of inpatients were demented. The care they required was no different to those of the paediatric wards: many relatives or domestic helpers came to help with feeding, washing, and other aspects of personal care. In coping with the increasing demands of dependent older people, there was increasing focus on duration of stay as a performance measure, giving rise to a 'revolving door' phenomenon.

We had a great team for care of the elderly in the New Territories East Cluster: we initiated many initiatives such as restraint reduction, falls prevention, use of technology and robots to aid rehabilitation, telemedicine to support residential care homes in the 1990s, and establishing liaison with many community NGOs. Yet we could not keep pace with demand, and the gap and dilemma of meeting the needs of such patients and what could actually be done rapidly widened.

In my personal life, both sets of family developed various age-related problems, requiring navigating though different health and social care systems, as well as social and psychological support. I approach these problems from a professional perspective, but have gradually realized how inadequate this is, in spite of the fact that geriatric medicine is supposed to provide holistic care covering not just physical health (how various body systems malfunction), but also functional (capabilities in independent living), social, psychological, and nutritional domains. I like to think that all this effort and experience is not in vain. Working in a predominantly institutional environment narrows one's view on ageing and makes it very negative. In reality, people use hospital services in the last years of life, and the change in hospital service profile is a result of increasing life expectancy to approaching 100. The health discourse has been dominated by the Hospital Authority services; yet with population ageing, it is increasingly necessary to design or build on existing community services, using an integrated approach to cover both social and health needs to tackle various problems before people end up in hospitals, and also to support them after discharge, in the inexorable journey towards end of life. We are far from doing this; yet if we ignore or fail to understand the full spectrum of consequences of population ageing, public health expenditures will increase, while unmet needs will also continue to increase.

The United Nations has declared 2020–2030 to be a decade of healthy ageing, with many countries supporting this aspiration. Currently many indicators of health ageing and service models are being promoted. In many ways this approach covering the whole life course is a very positive aspect to tackling ageing. Central to this approach is the concept of empowerment. People need to understand how ageing affects their brain function, as well as physical capabilities, and not view ageing through the black and white lens of whether you have a disease or not. There is no drug that prevents these changes; however, there are many things one can do individually, and collectively as a society, that can contribute to delaying dependency for as long as possible. This book talks about some of these aspects, emphasizing that in the last analysis, we need to take charge of our own ageing.

The contents cover the current concept of healthy ageing, whether we are achieving healthy ageing in Hong Kong or not, the importance of social determinants of healthy ageing and social justice, and what we can do better, as well as what other countries are doing. My personal views may be unfamiliar to many people, yet I have found more resonance from many ordinary older people I talk to, as well as from dialogue with international communities. It is in the spirit of stimulating a change in paradigm of how we view ageing that this book is written. I believe that changes in mindset may be achieved by more and more people expressing what they need and grouping together to create a society that is truly age-friendly and that allows older adults to function in a meaningful way, whatever chronic diseases or disabilities that they may suffer from. Our future is in our own hands.

Chapter One

WHAT IS HEALTHY AGEING?

*T*he term 'healthy ageing' was not in my vocabulary for a large part of my professional career as a doctor. Patients are either healthy, or have diseases which may or may not be cured or controlled with medicines. When faced with someone for whom no drug treatment is available and who is dying, one feels powerless to help and tends to be disengaged. There are so many new developments in diagnostic procedures and drug developments that one needs to keep up to date with, as well as protocols and guidelines for whatever institution one works in. Yet death is inevitable, and with population ageing, many people who are in hospital are facing death. Doctors should help them confront death, by first coming to terms with their own mortality. Later in my career when I had to deal with patient complaints, one patient wrote: 'There is a doctor that comes round every morning in the ward that I am in, to do a ward round. I know there is no cure for me, but I wish he would look at me and talk to me, instead of just looking at my charts at the end of the bed.'

When I started looking after older patients in 1985, it gradually occurred to me that values for measurement of older patients were not within normal limits, according to the normal ranges provided for the general population. Some of the older people would have been classified as having a disease using the latter measurement. Such observations and subsequent studies showed that we need to distinguish between age-related changes and diseases. The management for each is quite different. Furthermore many 'evidence based' treatments had been based on randomized controlled trials which do not reflect real life situations. There are many practical implications: should one classify obesity using just one value? With age there are hormonal changes that result in changes in body shape *with increasing waist measurements. If we adopt this approach, then many people in their 70s and 80s will be labelled as obese and told to go on a diet.*

As a result of engaging in many community projects relating to older people, the importance of doctors, hospitals, drugs, and investigations began to take a less important role, while social determinants of health became more important in a holistic view of health. For example, 40% of dementia is preventable through modification of lifestyle and air pollution. Social isolation and loneliness are medical, and indeed public health issues. If the health impact is as great as cigarette smoking, why is public health legislation somewhat unbalanced?

From a personal point of view, what does healthy ageing mean to me? Why are some people so active well into their 90s, while some become dependent on others for care for many years before they die? Many of us would agree that the first option would be preferable. So health is not just the absence of disease. Our paradigm of healthy ageing also needs to change, to adapt to the likelihood of people living to 100 years old.

●   ●   ●

Many people think that ageing is something that happens to others, while dying or depending on others for help in daily self-care activities are distant events that are best left for the future. This is especially true in the absence of any serious illnesses. Medical students learn about disease diagnosis, pharmacological or surgical treatments, with an emphasis on technological advancements. Doctor consultations seldom consist of how one should deal

Fig. 1.1 The life course approach to healthy ageing

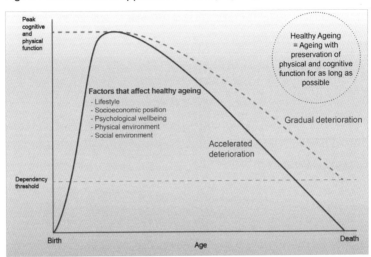

with age-related changes *per se*, independent of diseases. Yet these changes by themselves may result in the need to rely on other people as a result of a decline in brain and physical function.

We reach peak brain and physical function between 20–30 years of age. After that there is steady deterioration, which may not be noticeable at first, but is more obvious later on (Fig. 1.1). For example, you may notice that you cannot keep up with the pace of walking with people who are much younger, like your children or grandchildren. Yet it is possible to slow down these age-related changes through our own efforts. To a large extent, it is up to each of us to optimize our lifestyle, as well as advocating for a physical and social environment that enables us to do so. This goal is best expressed as healthy ageing, a term that is promoted by the World Health Organization (WHO) for 2020–2030 as the Decade of Healthy Ageing (WHO, 2020). Ageing societies where healthy ageing occurs are likely to have less burden in terms of need for medical and long-term care services.

Hong Kong currently has the longest life expectancy in the world, being 83.2 and 87.9 years for men and women, respectively. Is Hong Kong achieving the goal of healthy ageing at the same time? What this involves goes beyond disease prevention and management, but takes centre stage in the Sustainable Development Goals (SDGs).

Furthermore, healthy ageing as a goal involves action throughout the life course, from childhood to adolescence, to working life through retirement. This approach promoted by the WHO is a very constructive view of the ageing process. In other words, what you do when younger will affect how you age. Individual and societal response should not adopt a narrow perspective and focus only on non-communicable diseases (NCDs) and avoiding death, but to have an ultimate goal of maintaining functional ability for as long as possible. Health should be considered from the perspective

Fig. 1.2 Contribution of sustainable development goals to healthy ageing

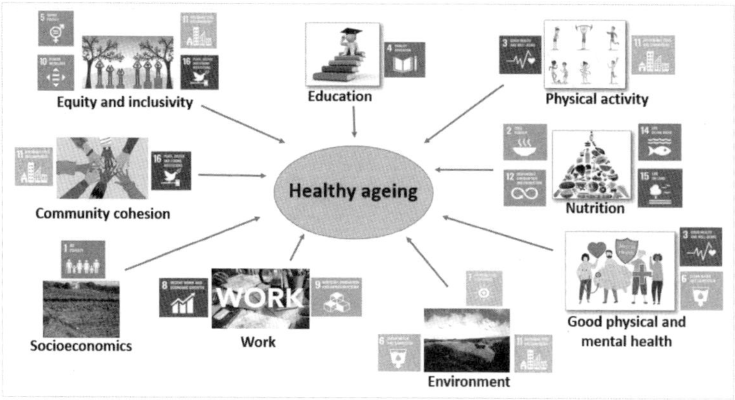

Adapted from Mavrodaris et al., 2022.

of an older person's functioning rather than the diseases at any one time, as well as all the external social and physical environments that may contribute to optimal functioning (Fig. 1.2). Inequities exist in healthy ageing and these should be addressed as part of social justice; therefore, tackling the social determinants of health forms an integral part of the response to ageing demographic changes. A key component consists of empowering older people to adapt and take an active part in shaping the challenges faced by individuals and society as a whole.

How Do We Measure Healthy Ageing?

Adoption of the UN resolutions of the Decade of Healthy Ageing by governments must be accompanied by a plan of action to improve the lives of older people, through collaborative networks. For example, in the UK, the UK Ageing Network (UKANet) works to better understand the biological mechanisms of ageing and their impact on human health; translate research findings into policy and practices; bring in older people, funders, and healthcare professionals in their research; and act as a voice for researchers on ageing. Collaborative networks like this, in ageing biology and clinical translation that are interdisciplinary—drawing from the social science, humanities, economics, biomedical and physical sciences, and members of the public with lived experiences of ageing—provide a concrete example of what should be aspired to (Cox & Faragher, 2022).

Healthy ageing is intrinsically linked to sustainability and equity; yet there is a widespread view that places healthy ageing exclusively in the chronic disease domain, and often only from the service providers' perspective rather than the older person's perspective (Mavrodaris et al., 2022).

Whether countries have implemented the UN resolutions, and how successful such efforts are, can be shown in the use of suitable indicators of healthy ageing. Such indicators are different from existing health indicators such as mortality and disease incidence, prevalence, and disability. Metrics are currently being explored by the WHO that include a life course approach in measuring intrinsic capacity, and that capture five domains focusing on function as an outcome (sensory, locomotor, vitality, psychological, and cognitive functions) (Thiyagarajan et al., 2022). Since then, the WHO has developed a model of Integrated Care for Older People (ICOPE) using a person-centred approach to manage older people with declining intrinsic capacity and functional ability which are key to healthy ageing (Fig. 1.3).

Central to these indicators is the assessment of functional outcomes from the older person's perspective. Factors that modify these outcomes go beyond personal attributes and healthy lifestyle behaviours, to health services, housing, urban planning, safe neighbourhoods that promote social networks, as promoted by the Age-friendly Cities (AFC) concept (Fig. 1.4) (CUHKIOA, 2022b, 2022c, 2022d, 2022e).

The term 'functional ability' is often interpreted as a personal attribute (covered in the intrinsic capacity domain), describing whether individuals can look after themselves as well as participate in society independently. The WHO gives a broader definition, covering domains such as the ability to meet basic needs, to learn, grow and make decisions, to be mobile, to build and maintain relationships and to contribute. Items under each

Fig. 1.3 The WHO's ICOPE

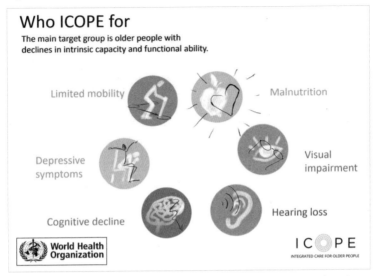

Source: World Health Organization. https://www.who.int/teams/maternal-newborn-child-adolescent-health-and-ageing/ageing-and-health/integrated-care-for-older-people-icope.

Fig. 1.4 Domains of Healthy Ageing

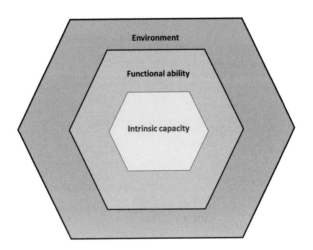

domain are broad, and very much from an individual's perspective rather than from the service providers' perspective. As such these cut across several disciplines and service providers, showing that an integrated approach is needed. For example, the ability to meet basic needs include being able to afford an adequate diet, clothing, suitable housing, health care, and long-term care.

Data that includes these indicators need to be collected on a regular basis to monitor trends, as well as the effectiveness of healthy ageing policies. Currently such data are not collected in regular surveys; only those related to mortality and causes of death are collected. The WHO is currently constructing a list of indicators based on validated tools to measure intrinsic capacity and functional ability, with the input of various expert advisory groups (Thiyagarajan et al., 2022).

This perspective underscores how important it is that older individuals take ownership of these issues that are important in maintaining their functional ability, and to ensure that there is adequate societal response.

Older people themselves have a crucial role to play, both in advocating for the need for relevant healthy ageing outcomes by participating in collaborative groups such as that in the UK described above, as well as ensuring that such indicators are included in regular government surveys (Fig. 1.5). We should move beyond being passive recipients of healthy ageing messages that are not accompanied by any societal changes that promote healthy ageing.

Fig. 1.5 Citizen participation for healthy ageing

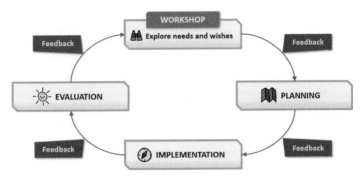

Chapter Two

ARE WE ACHIEVING HEALTHY AGEING IN HONG KONG?

*I*t is good that there are so many databases that rank various performance measures between countries, and between institutions. Behavioural insights show that people responsible take notice and aspire to move up rankings. University rankings are a great example and definitely drive how universities are run and their funding sources. If total life expectancy (TLE) at birth is used as a measure of healthy ageing, Hong Kong will be number one in the world for both men and women. So there is nothing to aspire to! Indeed, this may explain why healthy ageing policies do not receive such high priorities compared with waiting lists for specialist consultations. Important officials have expressed a view that the current healthcare system is the best and most efficient in the world, contributing to the high TLE.

While TLE may be a reasonable indicator of healthy ageing in low- and middle-income countries, in developed countries or economies such as Hong Kong, TLE may not be a suitable indicator, since the essentially free healthcare system may just be fulfilling the function of delaying death. A better indicator would be health span, the number of years lived without physical or cognitive function impairment. The ratio of health span divided by lifespan would be a better indicator of healthy ageing in developed economies. Such data is not collected regularly except through sporadic research projects. The nearest indicator is disability free life expectancy. These projects show that there is a trend towards increasing disability with time, with a gap of about ten years between men and women.

Since women have a longer TLE, the trend would be magnified by considering health span/life span. How do we care for this sector of the population? Over 20 years ago I asked the staff of a non-acute hospital to estimate how many hours of care are needed from nurses and/or personal care workers, for different levels of care, from their current experience. When this number was applied to residential care homes there was a huge difference, being greater in private homes. The profile of people being cared for are similar. Why should there be a difference in quality of standards of care? The COVID-19 pandemic put a spotlight on this neglected area that resulted in huge excess mortality for residents of old age homes during the circulation of the milder but more infectious Omicron variant.

Many years ago, in the course of a project inviting older adults who had fallen and attended Accident and Emergency Departments (AED) for further assessment, with subsequent referral to the geriatric clinic where I was seeing these patients, one patient was referred to me because she screened positive for depression. She lived in a residential care facility. When it was first opened she moved in with friends (originally classified as a hostel). With time they all died, and the residents were largely bedridden and could not talk. She went out every day, swimming and participating in activities of the nearby community centre. She fell because she was attempting to stand on one leg. She was not happy because she wanted to go out at night but the home did not allow her to go out. She wanted to move out but did not know where to go. As a doctor in the clinic, I felt totally irrelevant and unable to help. One thing is clear: drug treatment for depression would be inappropriate.

I saw an 80-year-old woman in the geriatric outpatient clinic, who had waited many months for the appointment. She had chest pain mainly at night, an abdominal hernia (a protrusion of the abdominal contents), back pain (was told she had osteoporosis), knee pain, had fallen a few times as her legs gave way, and lived alone after the recent death of her son. She was referred to the Cardiac Clinic in the first instance, but appropriately the referral was directed to the Geriatric Clinic. Her other outpatient appointments were Orthopaedic (for osteoporosis and knee pain presumably) and Surgical (abdominal hernia). The Geriatric Clinic appointment was the first of the three that she had to wait over a year for. So in desperation she went to the AED, since she thought that she may well have died of heart disease or broken many bones while waiting for the Cardiac and Orthopaedic Clinics. She was there from 2 pm and left after about 10 pm, after being seen by a doctor and told to wait for the results of the ECG, because from her perspective no one had helped her and she was very cold. She was given a packed dinner while waiting.

A quick assessment in the Geriatric Clinic established that the history was more compatible with symptoms of a hiatus hernia; that the abdominal hernia was diffuse due to generalized weakness of the abdominal wall muscles and although easily reducible, did affect her activities in the upright posture; that she had osteoarthritis affecting the knees; that she had mild kyphosis (an abnormally excessive convex curvature of the spine) likely from osteoporotic vertebral collapse; that she had reactive depression from the loss of her adult son; that she was worried about finances; and last of all she thought she was better off dead since the government did not seem to care and maybe deliberately made the waiting lists so long that elderly people would die quicker. She commented that the government looks after new immigrants better than old people like her, and cited in detail the total allowances that can be given out to a family of four of approximately $20,000 per month. She stated that there will never be any equality in our society except in death. She exhibited a fascinating mixture of having cognitive impairment in some aspects and very clear thinking on some issues. The above stories illustrate *older people's experience in the community, regarding unmet needs that extend beyond the disease paradigm.*

•   •   •

Hong Kong has a growing ageing population (see Fig. 2.1 below). This changing demography results from the falling fertility rate together with increasing total life expectancy at birth, following global patterns. For example, since 1960, the world's total fertility rate has halved while global life expectancy increased from 48 to 72 years. Increasing prevalence of non-communicable diseases accompanying this demographic change puts pressure on health and social care systems, with increasing medical, formal and informal care costs. Another consequence is the loss of productivity due to non-communicable diseases, which has

Fig. 2.1 Population of Hong Kong aged 65 and above and below 18 (1993–2018)

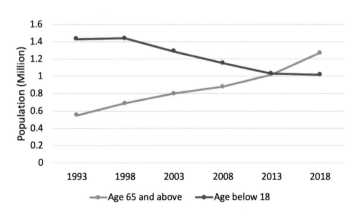

Source of data: Census and Statistics Department, HKSAR Government, 2019.

been estimated to range from 3% to 10% of GDP annually in the United States (Bloom, 2022). Older people consume more resources than they produce; hence the need to increase the rate of savings with increasing age. This demographic change has been described as a 'slow burning catastrophe' for societies that are unprepared for it, particularly the economic consequences. An investment in life-long health is needed to ensure that people may extend their working life, with consequent mental and physical health benefits (The Lancet Healthy Longevity, 2022).

There is a need to take a multi-disciplinary approach, to include not just health, but also social, economic, and policy aspects. It would be pertinent to examine the Hong Kong situation using the World Health Organization's healthy ageing lens.

Social Aspects

This is sometimes represented as the elderly dependency ratio from the economic viewpoint, assuming that older people reaching retirement age are economically inactive, and that they are supported by younger people who are in active employment. This concept may not be entirely applied to Hong Kong, since retirement at a certain age is not immutable, and there are examples of people who only retire when their health does not allow them to continue working, such as doctors in the private sector, musicians, and writers. With retirement and loss of income, poverty among older people increases. The poverty indicator used is the percentage of people with an income that is 50% below the population median. Using this definition, 549,000 (44.9%) people aged 65 and above live in poverty in Hong Kong (HKSAR, 2020). However, this does not take into account sources of income from investments, property rental income, family support, or various government means tested social allowances or universal benefits such as transport discounts. What is important is whether one has enough money to live on, which depends on their area of residence and lifestyle. When this question is included in a survey of people aged 60 years and above living in the community in five districts of Hong Kong sampled across a broad range of socioeconomic attributes, adequacy of disposable income had a stronger association with self-rated health. The absolute income corresponding to what is considered adequate lies between HKD 4,000 and 10,000 per month (Woo et al., 2020). Currently there is no good poverty indicator for the retired population.

Economic Impact

The economic consequence of increasing dependency has not been documented in Hong Kong, other than isolated papers from academia. A study of 1,820 older people living in a representative sample of residential care facilities over ten years ago already showed that an approximate estimation of staff numbers required for care based on a case-mix of residents' profiles showed considerable understaffing for non-subvented homes (Woo & Chau, 2009). A later study showing increasing trends in physical dependency and cognitive impairments over ten years showed how staff shortage problems could be accentuated due to increasing dependency of residents, with important implications for quality of care (Yu et al., 2019). Similarly, the quality of care for dependent older adults has not received much attention, in spite of the availability of assessment tools that guide care pathways. At regular intervals in the past 40 years, 'scandals' have been reported in the newspapers about poor treatment of older dependent adults, such as a group of naked residents being hosed down on the rooftop as a method of showering. Use of restraints to prevent falls and for people with dementia are common practice in long-term care.

Health Services

In Hong Kong, older adults are major users of hospital services. Older adults aged 65 and above account for 62% of general outpatient attendance, 56% of specialist outpatient attendance, 50% of patient bed days, and 89% of community nursing services (Yeoh & Lai, 2016) (Table 2.1).

This is partly because the driver of the use of hospital inpatient services is proximity to death rather than age per se (Woo, Goggins, et al., 2010). With an increase in life expectancy to 90 years, the number of people in hospital over the age of 80 will also increase. This is reflected in a change in the age profile of hospital inpatients in the past 40 years or so.

Table 2.1 Health status for elderly in Hong Kong

Chronic Diseases		Frailty		
None	More than one	Robust	Pre-frail	Frail
30%	70%	35%	52%	13%

Source of data: Census and Statistics Department. *Thematic Household Survey Reports* No. 40 and No. 58., Aug 2009 and Oct 2015; Woo et al., 2015.

There is no inequality in access to hospital services since these are free for those who receive Comprehensive Social Security Assistance (CSSA). In fact, those who are on CSSA use services slightly more frequently (Fig. 2.2) (Chung et al., 2021).

People with chronic diseases are major users of health services. The prevalence of chronic diseases increases among older people. Estimating the burden of these diseases, economic costs and impact on quality of life require data on trends in the rate of onset of a disease (incidence), as well as the case fatality rate. A

Fig. 2.2 Average number of AED visits during the last year of life, by CSSA status (2004–2014)

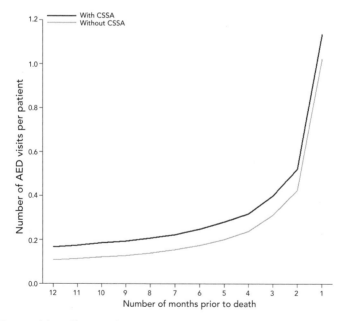

Source of data: Chung et al., 2021.

combination of high incidence and low fatality rate will result in the greatest burden, represented by the prevalence (Chan et al., 2013). For example, for 2010 the number of people aged 65 years and above with stroke was estimated to be 60,000, with 20,000 requiring residential care. By 2036 the numbers are projected to be 160,000 and 50,000, respectively. The direct medical cost of stroke for older people aged 65 years and above is estimated to be HKD 1.5 billion in 2010 and projected to increase to HKD 4.0 billion in 2036. The indirect cost of informal care is even higher, at HKD 5 billion to HKD 13.3 billion.

Corresponding figures for dementia are even higher, at HKD 228 billion increasing to HKD 594 billion. There are indications that public health services are already stretched to the limit; the waiting times for stable new cases booking at Specialist Outpatient clinics (1 April 2022 to 31 March 2023) ranged from nine weeks for Paediatrics to 216 weeks for Ophthalmology (Hospital Authority, 2023). Waiting at Accident and Emergency Departments may reach over eight hours, depending on the urgency of the complaint. This was magnified during the fifth wave of the COVID-19 pandemic, when dependent older people were shown in the media in beds on the pavement outside hospitals.

In the absence of chronic diseases, the ageing process itself also results in changes that predispose to declining physical and cognitive function, which may ultimately lead to dependency as well as increase in the use of health services. Such age-related changes may be grouped under the umbrella of geriatric syndromes such as frailty and sarcopenia (muscle loss). For example, frailty increases the risk of falls, disability, hospitalisation, and nursing home care, as well as mortality. Multimorbidity, frailty and disability singly and in combination have adverse impacts on health outcomes and increase the use of various types of healthcare services. The presence of all three conditions may increase risk of hospital admissions and outpatient attendances by 2.5 to 6.4-fold (Cheung et al., 2018).

The falling mortality trends from common NCDs in Hong Kong, together with an increasing total life expectancy at birth, suggests that the former is a major contributor, and hence prevention and management of NCDs should take centre stage in promoting healthy ageing (Ni et al., 2021). Such public health efforts, while successful, have pushed back but not eliminated these diseases, which appear at a later stage in life when age-related changes become more prominent; and an integrated medical, social and environmental approach is needed, as expressed in the WHO document ICOPE.

Ageist Attitudes

The public's perception of what being old means is very much shaped by media. Being old equates with having chronic diseases, being poor, and making no further contribution to society, which is a very negative image of being marginalized to the point of stigmatisation (Figs. 2.3–2.4).

An example of this was provided during the refurbishment of a ground-floor kindergarten in a public housing estate into a one-stop community centre for older people. Complaint letters were sent to government bodies: one letter asked the centre to provide data regarding how syringes were to be handled (the

Fig. 2.3 Negative images of ageing

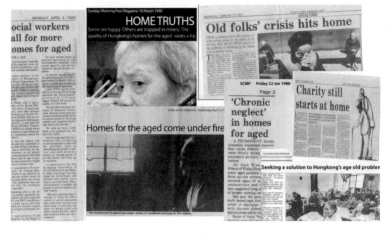

Fig. 2.4 Examples of ageism

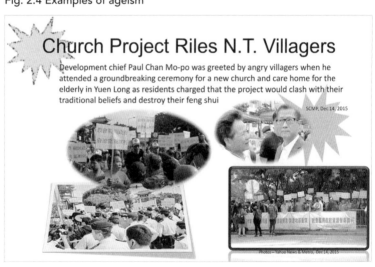

centre was not even a clinic). One district councillor actually coordinated a demonstration outside distributing pamphlets encouraging residents to object to the government. Subsequently residents complained that the air-conditioning units blew out hot air, which affected passers-by, even though the units were well above their heads. It is doubtful whether such complaints would be made if the site was used as a kindergarten again.

The negative stereotyping that gives rise to these examples shows a steady increase from the beginning of the 20th century to now (Ng et al., 2015). There is a misconception that older people are respected and well taken care of among Chinese cultures—the concept of filial piety. Yet this phenomenon may no longer be applicable in modern economies. In fact, a worldwide comparative study showed that the strongest level of senior derogation existed in East Asia, compared with the US and Europe (Woo, 2020). Negative stereotyping portrays older people as a burden, and policies tend to ignore their needs. The COVID-19 pandemic put a spotlight on how the needs of older adults were not considered. Pandemic policies caused great hardships for those who needed rehabilitation after complex illness, end-of-life care, dementia day care, and vaccination policies. Many of these services were shut down. Marked functional and cognitive deterioration were documented. In reality such services are just as needed as outpatient clinics or hospital beds, and should have been classified as essential. Older people themselves need to have a voice to state their needs, instead of needing to go to the private sector, which is not affordable by many.

There is health inequality in that those who can afford it can have better care in terms of their ability to employ personal helpers at home, to pay for residential care with better staff ratios and physical environments, and to use long-stay private hospitals. The burden of care largely rests on family members, with little support from society. Reported cases of murder-suicide attempts among elderly couples represent the tip of the iceberg for carer stress (Ho et al., 2009).

During the fifth wave of the COVID-19 pandemic at the beginning of 2022, outbreaks occurred in over 90% of residential care homes for the elderly, with 5,000 deaths between February and May, representing the highest death rate per million population worldwide. The physical environment of RCHEs, staff shortages, the frail profile and poor nutrition status of residents, vaccine hesitancy, and lack of a co-ordinated policy for integrated care for older people all contributed (Woo, 2022a).

The WHO report on ageism (WHO 2021) emphasizes that no sector of the population should be disadvantaged according to chronological age. It seems that Hong Kong still has some way to go in achieving this objective, and growing voices from older people themselves will be critical in counteracting ageism and ensuring that all policies are formulated through a non-ageist lens.

These descriptions are all the more perplexing, since we all age. Perhaps there is a collective societal denial of inevitable decline, as a result of the majority of individuals having bad experiences of ageing. On the other hand, putting a focus on all the positive aspects, banning the use of 'age discriminatory words' such as 'elderly' and 'frail', may equally be another aspect of denial. These sentiments are particularly strong in Western societies. It is important to have a balanced view, seeking to understand what happens as one gets older, and to develop personal strategies to prepare for the likely occurrence of the 100-year life. We should make sure that policies are there to facilitate these strategies. This represents true empowerment, and an opportunity to 'take charge of our own ageing'.

Chapter Three

IS SOCIAL INEQUALITY
MAKING US SICK?

*T*he development of health services is heavily emphasized by what occurs in hospitals. Unfortunately, the evolution of health seen through the hospital lens, and also through innovative technologies, has widened the gap between what ageing people need and what is provided in terms of service design, availability, and implementation of responsive policies.

> 'Biomedicine has increasingly banished the illness experience as a legitimate object of clinical concern. Carried to its extreme, this orientation, so successful in generating technological inter-ventions, leads to a veterinary practice of medicine'. (Kleinman et al., 1978)

Although the ageing experience may not equate with the illness experience, it suffers the same neglect, in being relegated to a merely 'social' problem. Perhaps subconsciously the Hong Kong society values older people less, however it may be politically incorrect to state this explicitly. Consider this: in recent years summers are getting hotter, and the media have frequently reported on the plight of people living in cramped spaces in areas considered 'heat islands', and also public housing without air conditioning. It is known that extreme heat affects both physical and psychological health, increasing hospital admissions and suicide rates among older adults. Where is our community heat action plan other than issuing hot weather warnings? McDonald's may be commended on allowing people to stay 24 hours before pandemic policies removed this refuge. Racing horses are looked after better: racing is postponed to late afternoons and evenings during hot weather, with installation of cooling fans blowing out water as well. In Mediterranean countries working hours are amended to avoid the hottest part of the day, while buildings have *reflective shutters. In the public square in Bordeaux, there is a large area with holes in the ground that at intervals blow out a fine mist. By standing in the mist, one cools off with evaporation of the water. In Hong Kong we have similar devices except that they are used for watering roses in the Tai Po Waterfront Park.*

The creation of Age-friendly Cities is one of the factors promoting healthy ageing. In Hong Kong we have shown that indicators of an elder quality of life covering many domains, including the WHO Age-friendly Cities indicators, deteriorated during the year of social unrest followed by the COVID-19 pandemic (Woo et al., 2021). Clearly, health services are not able to influence these domains, but policies do. For example, the UK recently passed a law making it illegal for people to obstruct the roads (climate change activists were being targeted). If Hong Kong had enacted such a law, would 2019 have had such a huge impact on society? Did the pandemic policies contribute to the decline? Should policies only be enacted in terms of a definition of public health that is entirely based on the numbers of infected people and whether hospitals can cope? (Woo, 2022c).

● ● ●

There is a social gradient (as well as gender difference) in healthy ageing in Hong Kong. Should our society accept this? The social determinants of health have been widely documented in the past few decades, pointing out that health is not only determined by healthcare professional services and systems (Marmot et al., 2022). Health conditions may be improved by the healthcare system, only to be adversely affected if social determinants are ignored (Fig. 3.1). It has been argued that health equity is a matter of social justice,

Fig. 3.1 A balance between successful pandemic control and adverse consequences for older people

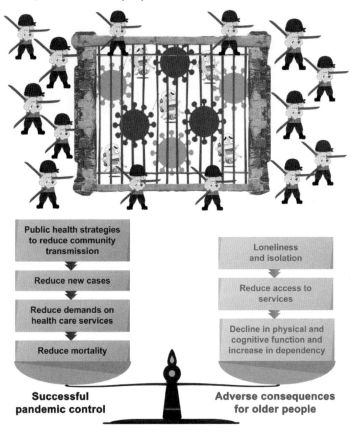

and this goal should be a recurrent theme in all policies, given that social determinants cover a wide range of situations where people grow up, live, work, and grow old throughout their life course. Health equity is not merely a reflection of income and status, and access to health services.

There are health inequalities among older adults using healthy ageing as an outcome measure, in addition to chronic disease indicators. Other than the increasing prevalence of non-communicable diseases as one becomes older, the occurrence of geriatric syndromes (which reflects the ageing process itself) becomes more common in extremes of old age. The latter requires an integrated medical and social response in the community setting, compared with the predominantly medical and hospital/clinic response for diseases (Fig. 3.2).

Fig. 3.2 Non-communicable diseases and geriatric syndromes at different ages

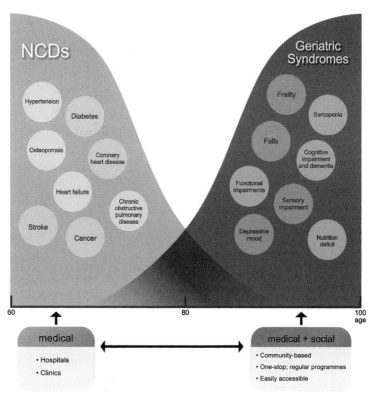

In Hong Kong, health inequalities for older adults exist at two levels.

Firstly, the needs of older people as a group are seldom considered separately from the general adult population in the formulation of health policies and guidelines. For example, despite the well acknowledged fact that Hong Kong is an ageing society, the indicator for Body-Mass Index (BMI) used by the Department of Health is still used for the general population, without a separate index for older people. As the need for older people is different, adhering to the general population standard will create confusion or, worse still, misconceptions that older people need to keep their weight low to fit the 'standard'. The COVID-19 pandemic policies also provide a spotlight on this issue. Vaccination policy and requirements for socialising were based on the assumption of computer literacy; community support and rehabilitation services after hospital discharge were halted in favour of dealing with acute COVID-19 cases; the inadequacies of care of very frail older adults in residential care homes were magnified, contributing to fatality rates from Omicron at the beginning of 2022 that were the highest in the world (Woo, 2021, 2022b). Some 5,000 older people in residential care homes died in this fifth wave, representing the majority of elderly deaths. Contrary to the popular narrative, this may not be explained entirely by suboptimal vaccination rates. Frailty, a suboptimal physical environment for containment of infectious diseases as well as a shortage of care staff all contributed. Subjective social status increases the risk of incident frailty in a 14-year follow-up study, independent of objective measures of social economic status, chronic diseases, unhealthy lifestyle, poor mental health and poor cognitive function (Yu, Tong, Leung, et al.,

2020). The district of residence also influences physical and mental quality of life, frailty, and mortality, independent of lifestyle factors and socioeconomic position, showing that where one lives impacts on health outcomes (Woo, Chan, et al., 2010). A study of Sha Tin and Tai Po districts found that older people who perceived their district as more age-friendly had better self-rated health (Wong, Yu et al., 2017). Frail men have more improvements living in districts with more green space, while residents of such districts will benefit from reduced risks of mortality (Wang, Lau et al., 2017). Perceived neighbourhood environment is related to self-rated health among community-dwelling older Chinese (Wong et al., 2017). Older people residing in districts with better neighbourhood social cohesion feel happier and have more life satisfaction and meaning in life (Yu et al., 2019).

Secondly, it is important to be aware of gender health inequalities especially among older adults (Fig. 3.3, Tables 3.1–3.3). In general, women live longer but spend more of their lives being dependent. Currently much of the discourse regarding gender inequalities is focused on attaining equality in positions of power, influence, and financial status, rather than health. There is consistent documentation of differences in life expectancies, disease prevalence and disease mortality, and geriatric syndromes such as frailty and sarcopenia.

Horizontal justice requires that there be equal treatment and benefits for equal needs of men and women, while vertical justice requires that there be differential treatment and benefits for differential needs of men and women. Gender-based inequalities over the life course in a sociocultural context exert a strong influence on healthy ageing.

Fig. 3.3 Gender differences in the trajectory of functional decline according to frailty groups

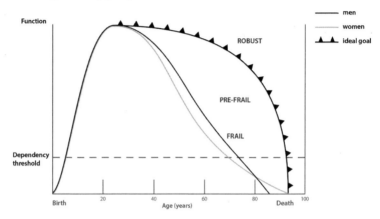

Indexes to track changes in well-being compiled by the CUHK Jockey Club Institute of Ageing from 2017 to 2020 reveal that compared with male counterparts, older women had a higher poverty rate, rated themselves poorer in health, had lower mental health and were frailer (Chau and Lee, 2022). Although women live longer than men, they spend a longer period in a frail state, have higher prevalence of depression (although the suicide rate is lower), musculoskeletal pain, higher prevalence of sarcopenia and faster rate of decline in muscle mass and physical performance measures, and higher prevalence of cognitive impairment. Underlying factors contributing to gender differences in healthy ageing include, biological, behavioural, socioeconomic, as well as cultural. For example, the caregiver role is frequently delegated to women, and this role confers a greater risk of depression and worse health (Ho et al., 2009). Higher self-ranking of community standing is associated with better health outcomes (Woo et al., 2008). In general women tend to adopt healthier lifestyles compared with men, and there is a sex difference in stress response, which affect health.

> **Sex Differences in Stress Responses**
> - 50 young adult healthy volunteers randomly assigned to social rejection or achievement stress conditions
> - Stress assessed by self-report and salivary cortisol
> - Men showed greater response to achievement challenges
> - Women showed greater response to social rejection challenges, which may contribute to the increased rates of affective disorders in women
>
> Source: Stroud et al., 2002.

Table 3.1 Gender differences in 9,056 community-dwelling Chinese men and women in Hong Kong—the E-health study

Men Worse	Women Worse
Subjective well-being	Frailty
Polypharmacy	Sarcopenia
Hospitalisation	Cognitive screening
Day care utilisation	Self-rated health (<80 years)
	Instrumental Activities of Daily Living (IADL) (≥80 years)

Source: Unpublished data from Jockey Club Community E-Health Care Project.

Table 3.2 Gender differences in social determinants of frailty

	Men	Women
Job hierarchy	+	−
Not enough money	+	+
Physical activity	+	+
Alcohol (protective)	+	−
Frequency of contact with relatives	−	+
Number of relatives	+	−
Number of neighbours	+	+
Help others	+	+
Attend community/religious activities	−	+

Source: Woo et al., 2005.

Table 3.3 Caregiver role. Multiple conditional logistic regression analysis on odds ratio of reporting symptoms, depression and worse health, comparing Primary Informal Caregivers (PCGs) with Noncaregivers (NCGs), stratified by sex

	Men (N=231)				Women (N=507)			
	PCG (N=77), %	NCG (N=154), %	Odds Ratio*	95% Confidence Interval	PCG (N=169), %	NCG (N=338), %	Odds Ratios*	95% Confidence Interval
Anxiety in the past 4 weeks	36.8	22.7	2.33	1.20–4.53	45.6	29.0	2.18	1.45–3.29
Depression (≥16)	23.4	14.3	2.36	1.09–5.09	24.3	10.4	3.19	1.81–5.60
Health compared with that 1 year ago, worse	35.1	24.7	1.96	1.01–3.80	37.9	23.4	2.44	1.55–3.84

*Adjusted for work status and educational levels.
Source: Ho et al., 2009.

Life Course Approach

A report on the life course approach to health inequalities in Hong Kong, compiled by the joint Institutes of Health Equity of the University College London (UCL) and CUHK, focuses on the social determinants of health that are key to explaining unfair differences in health according to social economic status. Social determinants such as education, occupation and housing affect the health of a person across life stages such as early childhood development, reading attainments, self-rated health and psychological distress among adolescents, working conditions and the stress of adults, which cumulatively affect well-being in their old age (Figs. 3.4–3.5). In Hong Kong, the infant mortality rate is among the lowest in the world due to the robust maternal and child health support system, but inequalities start to be observed in school readiness according to the socioeconomic status of the families of the children. It in turn affects the schools they will study at, academic performance, life satisfaction, self-rated health, and the chance of studying in universities. Upon transition to work, non-degree holders are paid less and are more likely to work in low-paying jobs with long working hours and vulnerable working conditions.

Stepping into old age, those disadvantaged will suffer from inadequate finances, more likelihood of depressive symptoms, and a higher level of frailty. While in Hong Kong the suicide rate for older people is the highest among different age groups, there is a socioeconomic gradient in suicide for older people (Fig. 3.6) (CUHKIHE, 2022).

Fig. 3.4 Stages of the life course and the accumulation of effects

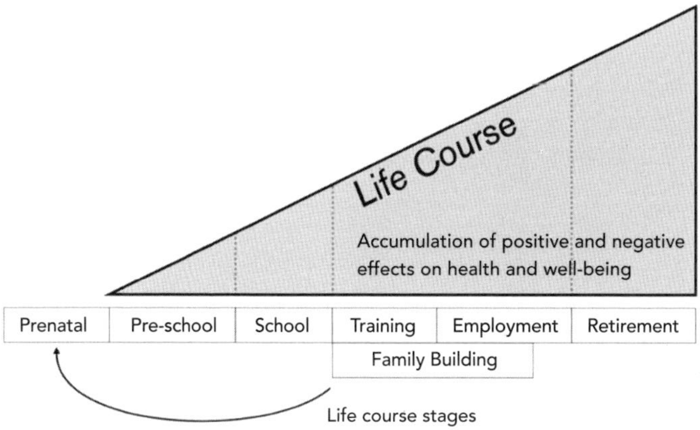

Source: CUHK Institute of Health Equity Report, 2022.

Fig. 3.5 Health inequalities in Hong Kong

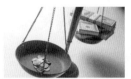

Socioeconomic inequalities will give rise to inequalities in health in later life

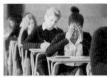

Young adults have high levels of psychological distress

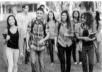

Problems for adolescents and university students have increased, related to the effects of the COVID-19 pandemic and social unrest

Long working hours worsen physical and mental health and increase inequalities

Loneliness will worsen, more older people living alone

Older people from lower socioeconomic backgrounds experience more chronic disease, higher rates of depression

Inequalities in reading attainment among more and less privileged children at age 15

Suicide rates among older people are much higher

Fig. 3.6 Suicide rates by age group in Hong Kong, 2011–2021*

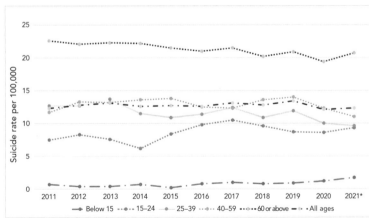

*Estimated number. According to data from the Coroner's Court, with registered death date up to 31 July, 2022.

It is important to monitor indicators of health inequality, and in the UK and US, health and social indicators according to areas of 'deprivation' have been collected as part of policies to address such inequalities. The concept of area of deprivation may not apply to Hong Kong, since it is a very densely populated city where there is no clear geographic demarcation between rich and poor districts. Instead, it may be more appropriate to use a measure of the number of people living in a certain area of floor space at home that is collected by the Hong Kong Census as an equivalent, as there is some evidence that living space is related to health outcomes (Chung et al., 2022).

A review by the World Health Organization found that individuals living in a crowded household have higher risks of infectious diseases and mental health problems. The result is echoed by local studies showing association of household crowding with adverse health outcomes such as hypertension, anxiety and stress in Hong Kong.

We need to adopt a biopsychosocial model of health that takes into account where we live and how we live. If increasing ambient temperature increases suicide rate in older adults, surely we should make every effort to devise community action plans to mitigate this impact. Likewise, loneliness and social isolation need to be recognised and dealt with as medical issues and not just social or mental health issues (Holt-Lunstad and Perissinotto, 2023), as they directly increase the risk of coronary heart disease, stroke mortality, dementia, susceptibility to infections, and dependency, in addition to anxiety and depression. These ultimately result in higher healthcare costs. The impact is as high as the traditional risk factors such as obesity or smoking. The UK, the US and various scientific and world health bodies have recommended policies to counter social isolation and loneliness. Hong Kong society has not recognised these as medical issues: indeed, pandemic policies created more isolation and loneliness, ironically in the name of public health.

Chapter Four

CAN WE DO BETTER?

We *have to do better, by realizing that currently, ten-year-old children can expect to live to 100 years and beyond. Societies need a paradigm shift to support the likely scenario of the 100-year life, with increasing age diversity. The metric of success is aligning health span with lifespan, taking into account working for longer and in more flexible ways, building financial security early on in life, and creating healthy communities that take into account built environments and urban planning resulting in better air quality and social spaces that promote social relationships. Unfortunately, many people in Hong Kong associate increasing lifespan in terms of increasing deficits and societal burden, thinking about older people as a distinct group and providing separate services. We need to re-imagine integrated health-promoting communities as described above instead.*

●　　●　　●

What are the strategies for achieving healthy ageing? Clearly, changes should not be confined to only the health domain, with a predominant focus on prevention, early detection and treatment of chronic individual diseases. Rather, a broader life course approach that includes the social determinants of health, with an awareness of age-related changes in addition to single diseases, should be adopted. The WHO's Report on healthy ageing in 2015, now widely promoted in the UN Decade of Healthy Ageing 2020–2030, could provide a blueprint to guide individuals and societies towards achieving this goal. This includes focusing on optimal development and preservation of intrinsic capacity, functional ability, and enabling physical and social environments. This response requires a paradigm shift for governments that formulate policies according to separate bureaus such as health, social welfare, urban planning, buildings, transport, leisure and culture, etc. Clearly, strong leadership with a clear vision of the challenges of population ageing will be needed to implement cross-sectoral responses effectively.

A Framework to Reduce Frailty Rates

The key to achieving healthy ageing lies in our own understanding of all the contributing factors and seeing how they apply to ourselves. This likely covers our own motivation to change behaviour related to adopting a health-promoting lifestyle as a habit, as well as examining the workplace, where we live, and social engagements. This approach is a radical departure from the current narrative of relying on doctors, investigations and drugs, accompanied by unrealistic expectations that bad health outcomes can be avoided if you do what the doctors tell you. The medical approach is focused on diseases: prevention, early detection and treatment. Resources for the medical system are already overwhelmed by these tasks. Yet we all need to understand how our bodily function changes with the ageing process itself, in order to maximise function and retard decline. This approach is no different to that for individual diseases: yet this aspect has not been systematically promoted, although the current community resource ecosystem is capable of providing a suitable infrastructure. However, the main driver has to be the older individuals themselves.

In the past decade or so, various initiatives in Hong Kong to raise health literacy and empowerment for older adults to understand age-related changes provide examples of how fruitful this approach

Fig. 4.1 Frailty and increased usage of health services

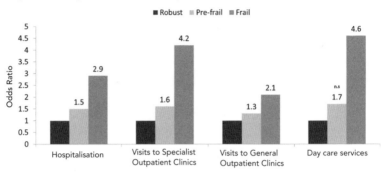

Source: Unpublished data from Jockey Club Community E-Health Care Project.

is, compared with the more paternalistic approach of the dominant medical narrative. Some of these are described below.

The concept of age-related decline in function, conceptualised under the term 'frailty' representing a loss of homeostatic mechanisms, has been promoted in the community in the past decade by the Jockey Club Institute of Ageing at the Chinese University of Hong Kong, supported by the Hong Kong Jockey Club Charities Trust. Frailty increases the utilisation of health services. To address this issue, a framework has been proposed as a model to be included in primary care for older adults (Figs. 4.1–4.2). This involves community screening, followed by a frailty prevention programme which runs for 12 weeks in groups of about ten participants each. In each session, they have exercises such as aerobic circuit training and resistance training; computer-assisted cognitive training, consisting of interactive touchscreen mini-video games to train cognitive domains of memory, attention, executive function, flexibility, and visuospatial ability; and board game activities to enhance interactions and friendships between participants. The programme has

Fig. 4.2 Multicomponent frailty prevention programme evaluation. The related study has been published in the *Journal of the American Medical Directors Association*

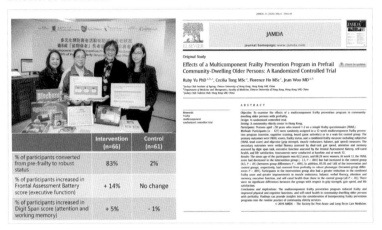

been shown to reduce frailty levels as well as improve cognitive function, and was developed and piloted in a community setting using a self-financed model (Figs. 4.3–4.5). Many people were very interested in the concept and in taking part in screening and lifestyle modification to prevent the development of frailty. Focus group findings essentially show that participants feel empowered to be in charge of their health without the use of medications, and that their habits have been changed because they feel so much better after participating in these programmes on a regular basis (Yu et al., 2021; Yu & So, et al., 2020; Yu & Tong et al., 2020).

We ran discussion groups for regular participants, who have stayed in the programme on a self-financing basis for up to seven years. This is an example of a group who participated in a community programme that is able to reverse or slow down age-related frailty just by changing their habits. Understanding how this behaviour change has been achieved is very important to driving other behaviour changes. One retired professional couple in their seventies said that they felt much healthier by coming regularly, and that they did not feel so good when they stopped. One participant commented that it is the whole physical environment of the Jockey Club Cadenza Hub (an initiative for seniors to promote positive ageing), where they feel that they can continue to learn about ageing issues in a place where they can check their own blood pressure, body mass index, and vision. 'It is not just arranging exercise classes', one of them said. Social groups have been formed, where members may continue with other activities that they arrange themselves, using knowledge acquired through various programmes relating to coping with age-related changes. One member shared how she had been discharged from hospital, and had no confidence in going out and participating in any social or physical activities. After joining the programme, she was able to go travelling with her family outside of Hong Kong.

Repeatedly there were questions of why there were not more such centres all over Hong Kong. This is an example of where behaviour change has been achieved that is important for the goal of maintaining function, or healthy ageing as defined in the broad sense by the World Health Organization. Participants assumed that this is being supported by the Charities Trust and run by the Chinese University of Hong Kong; in reality, the goal is an entirely self-financing operation, which is difficult to attain since rental is high. We introduced the concept of co-creation of a viable business model with members. Unfortunately, the pandemic and lack of manpower stopped this development. It is pertinent to ask why government outpatient clinics and hospitals do not pay any rent. Can such centres operate rent free? This would go a long way to facilitating the opening of similar centres in many vacant government premises, using a self-financing model. Perhaps community members can actively participate in its operation together with NGOs. This may be the future for the 100-year lifespan and, hopefully, health span.

Fig. 4.3 Impact of frailty intervention programme on frailty in older people

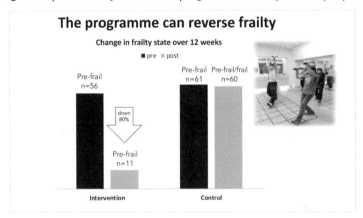

Fig. 4.4 Impact of frailty intervention programme on cognitive function of older people

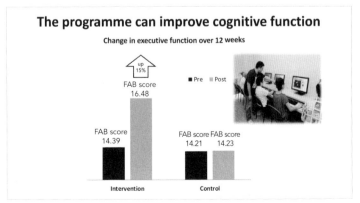

Fig. 4.5 High level of sustainability of the frailty intervention programme

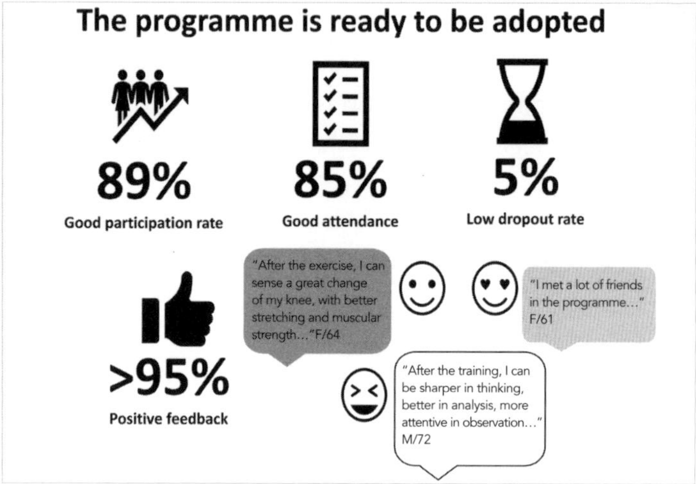

Technology Supporting Empowerment

With ageing, older adults encounter many problems that are not directly related to the presence of chronic diseases but to ageing processes themselves. Examples are problems with seeing, hearing, memory, lack of energy, falls, and reduced capacity to lift heavy objects or manage stairs. These are some of the manifestations of frailty and sarcopenia. It is important to understand the underlying reasons for such changes in order to take appropriate measures to retard decline. Self-screening, or screening administered by informal carers, may allow identification of problems earlier and facilitate appropriate action. This may involve further detailed assessment of cognitive function, guidance to various group programmes such as the frailty prevention programme described above, or to further information relating to management of abnormalities.

The E-health and E-tool projects carried out by the Jockey Club Institute of Ageing use automated methods for screening commonly encountered conditions under the intrinsic capacity domains of the WHO ICOPE programme. Through the use of a tablet or mobile app, older adults can assess their health situation with immediate results and targeted information for improvement. The E-health screening represents the first step in a step-care approach towards action, which may be designed in future with reference to available neighbourhood facilities. The E-tools screening consists of an app that covers similar domains, with directions to videos about the particular condition and management.

A Self-screening App For Older Adults

- A free self-help health screening mobile application
- Designed for older adults to perform health screening independently, at anytime, anywhere
- Homepage showcases 11 screening assessments, including: Frailty, Risk of Sarcopenia, Nutrition, Memory, Dental Health, Functional Ability, Self-caring, Incontinence, Hearing ability, Eyesight, Emotional Health, with simple icons to enhance understanding.
- After screening, test results, education materials, community resources and a comprehensive health report will be provided.

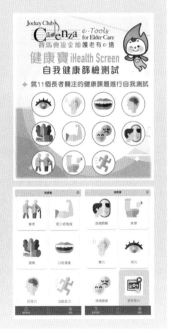

Promotion of the E-tools app, together with the accompanying education materials, has received enthusiastic responses from the public as well as formal and informal caregivers. The point is that the E-tools app fulfils some unmet needs and has been developed for the purpose of helping ourselves with ageing and caring issues. Paid carers of older people, whether in residential, day care or home settings, will be more competent in dealing with various problems that are commonly encountered, have a better understanding of underlying causes, and know where to turn to for help. For family members, such knowledge may reduce stress and reduce visits to doctors or hospitals. Various organisations have considered using E-tools as training for staff or volunteers. There is much room for development as an empowering tool. For example, by adding a GPS function, one can locate nearby health or social services. We already have this technology on our mobile phones and can locate the nearest McDonalds or Japanese restaurant. Is this not an example of a low-hanging fruit in our development of 'Gerontechnology'?

Shaping Our Neighbourhoods and Cities

According to the WHO framework on healthy ageing, the physical and social environments in which we live and work are important contributors. We can shape our neighbourhoods through greater understanding of the environment in which we live through the lens of the eight domains of the WHO's Age-friendly Cities (Fig. 4.6). More work is required, but some notable areas to make a more age-friendly Hong Kong are building an inclusive built environment, combating ageism, making information more accessible for older

Fig. 4.6 Domains of an Age-friendly City

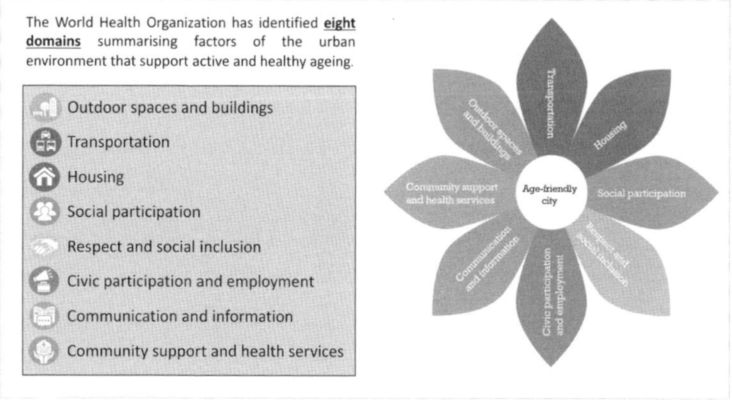
The World Health Organization has identified **eight domains** summarising factors of the urban environment that support active and healthy ageing.
Outdoor spaces and buildings
Transportation
Housing
Social participation
Respect and social inclusion
Civic participation and employment
Communication and information
Community support and health services
Transportation
Housing
Outdoor spaces and buildings
Community support and health services
Age-friendly city
Social participation
Communication and information
Civic participation and employment
Respect and social inclusion

people, creating a more inclusive labour market, and empowering the elderly to take care of their own health, to name a few. More details can be found in the *Age-friendly City Guidebook* published by the Institute of Ageing at CUHK, which has crystalised the experience of the project with practical guidance and resources for AFC development in Hong Kong (CUHKIOA, 2021a).

Taking the 'outdoor spaces and buildings' domain as an illustration, the current discourse of relying on universal design guidelines has totally missed the mark of being elderly friendly. To cater for the needs of older people, the Institute of Ageing at CUHK, with other parties, has been advocating for change through a series of interactive workshops accompanied by tours to various sites in Hong Kong focused on the interaction between health and urban and building design, and how older adults can contribute to advocacy in creating more enabling living environments. To empower older people to voice their views and needs, a pioneer work called the Nutcrackers Project (https://www.ioa.cuhk.edu.

hk/nutcrackers/index.html) has been set up to bring together the efforts of health and built environment practitioners, retirees, and students (Fig. 4.7). It uses the figurative image of digging for 'pine nuts' in Hong Kong, which are some attentive observations in the city where design can be further explored to help build quality environments in which Hong Kong people will be happy and safe to live.

Older people living in areas of Hong Kong that are less dense and in close proximity with open spaces (Figs. 4.8–4.9) compared with those in dense urban areas (Fig. 4.10) have a less-frail profile (CUHKIOA, 2022f). Perhaps many of the outlying islands or more rural areas could be sites for 'senior living' accommodations instead of relocation to mainland China areas, since medical support would not be an issue.

Fig. 4.7 Official website of the Nutcrackers Project

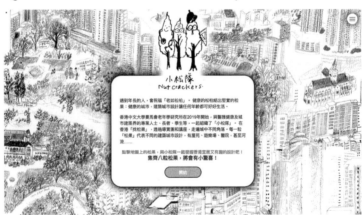

Fig. 4.8 Gathering of elders at an open area on Peng Chau

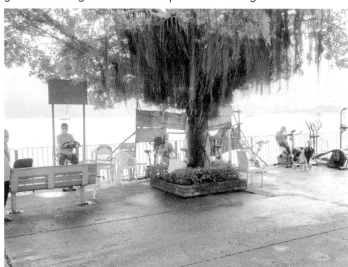

Fig. 4.9 Open area and shared facilities on Peng Chau

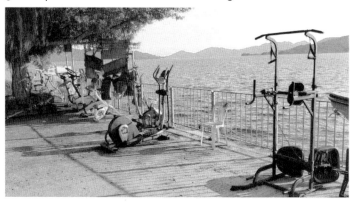

Fig. 4.10 Dense and tall buildings in Hong Kong

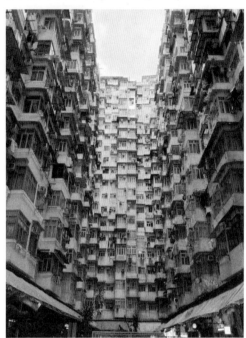

End-of-Life Choices

Other than not knowing how to control how we live, the fact that we can also control how we die is not commonly known. Healthy ageing ideally ends with a 'good death'. There is common consensus that this involves avoiding suffering, particularly pain, being in control of the environment in which death occurs, having sufficient time to prepare, and getting one's affairs in order (Meier et al., 2016). There is a misconception that there is a cure for all diseases, when in reality for the majority of diseases, medicine seldom provides a cure but merely helps patients to live with the condition, with the aim of maintaining optimal physical and cognitive function in the context of optimising quality of life. The trajectory of various chronic diseases towards death vary, being faster with most cancers compared with obstructive pulmonary diseases and heart failure, and longer with neurodegenerative diseases such as dementia. There are indicators of the proximity of death, such as the number of hospital admissions within a one-year period, together with the number of chronic diseases, which would provide a time frame for when it might be appropriate to start discussions with family and healthcare professionals, to express a choice of essentially comfort care versus prolonging the dying process.

While working as Honorary Chief of Service in Shatin Hospital about 15 years ago, we started an initiative to extend care of people at the end of life to those in the end stage of various chronic diseases, in addition to those with cancer. Some had reached the end stage of dementia and were not able to swallow food or drink. The question arises whether these patients should be fed using a nasogastric tube, to avoid starving to death. A tube is inserted through the nose to the stomach and taped to the face. Not uncommonly, patients pull it out because it is uncomfortable. Then their hands are tied down. They may still feel hungry and want to eat. The thinking is that tube feeding may reduce aspiration of food into the lungs and cause pneumonia. However, patients may still have aspiration pneumonia from aspirating saliva, or regurgitated stomach contents. Often careful handfeeding provides relatives with the last channel of communicating care and love to their relatives. Two daughters with the mother dying of dementia opted not to use the nasogastric tube, and took turns feeding their mother with food she liked. After her death, they articulated very well how this process enabled them to be with the mother, to feel that they were doing something to express care and love. As part of an education programme, they agreed to speak at a press conference. Afterwards the hospital switchboard was flooded with calls from people who wanted to be admitted to Shatin Hospital.

Most people want to know and prepare for proximity to death. During the last year or so, a person dying would want to get their affairs in order and have a say in treatment with discussion with family members. In particular, one may wish to avoid treatment that merely prolongs the dying process. Clearly, the beginning of this process starts with doctors, who have the responsibility to present a complete picture and not avoid the prospect in the name of not depriving the patient and family of hope. Usually, experienced doctors are more competent. Yet junior doctors are in contact with patients and their families more. As mentioned before, with changing population demographics, many older patients spend their last years in hospitals. Communications regarding end-of-life care should be a universal skill. Likewise, lay people need to understand chronic disease trajectories and details of management, and be empowered to make choices. In the past seven years, supported by the Jockey Club Charities Trust, the Institute of Ageing has been engaged in such an initiative: to empower patients, families and the general public, as well as raising competence in health and social care professionals in discussing end-of-life care issues.

How to initiate such serious illness conversations with healthcare professionals and family members, and how to record your wishes regarding end-of-life care in the form of advance care planning (ACP) and advance directive (AD), is also promoted by the Institute. Realistic videos of the terminal stages of chronic diseases and invasive treatment procedures are created, so that all may understand what receiving life-prolonging treatment actually involves, and what the alternatives are (Fig. 4.11). It may not be assumed that by default everyone would opt for life prolongation at any cost. In reality, a number of patients, particularly with chronic obstructive pulmonary diseases, would opt for comfort care rather than repeated mechanical ventilation. Their choice can be documented and should be respected by the healthcare team and family members. A good understanding of such choices may influence the episodic demands from the public for euthanasia and inform such debates.

Fig. 4.11 Educational videos on Heart Failure and Chronic Obstructive Pulmonary Disease (COPD). Examples of educational videos for the general public include 'Treatment options for heart failure' and 'Treatment options for COPD'. Both videos have received 323 and 381 views, respectively (as at 10 Jan 2023)

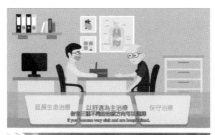
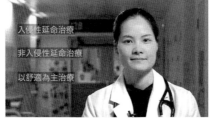

Family members, as well as some healthcare professionals, tend to avoid frank discussions; yet feedback from the public in general and from patients show wide interest in expressing their end-of-life wishes. The Institute of Ageing has, over the past few years, conducted interactive family sessions on advance care planning for patients and their family members recruited from various public hospitals (Fig. 4.12). The aims of the sessions include allowing the participants to understand the concepts and treatment options in end-of-life care and, more importantly, empowering and motivating them to take the leading role in initiating the communication process in advance care planning. In other words, participants are not considered passive beneficiaries, and they are not simply asked to blindly sign the advance directive in a mechanical manner. Instead, they are enabled to engage in discussions, and to actively think about and share their preferences in this regard.

Fig. 4.12 ACP family sessions at Shatin Hospital. Nineteen sessions were held (from 4 March 2021 to 8 December 2022), with 121 caregivers (of 72 patients), 3 medical colleagues and 2 nurses. Six patients signed ACP or AD voluntarily after the sessions

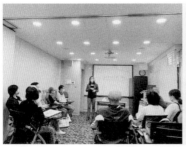
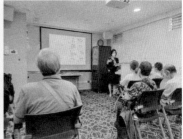

One session with patients and family members and staff of a non-acute hospital was particularly moving. Participants shared their thoughts and some cried. One patient with stroke started to express his wishes to his brother, while some regretted their choice of life-prolonging treatment for their relative, since they had not discussed this beforehand. An interesting observation was that most family members would not choose life-prolonging treatment for themselves. However, when asked whether they would choose it for their parents if something suddenly happened, inexplicably, most people agreed they would. This is a scenario that could be avoided by early discussion in the form of advance care planning.

In addition to patients and their family members, the Institute of Ageing has also conducted similar sessions for community-dwelling older people, and even the younger generations. Given that planning about end-of-life issues should be a revisable and ongoing process that is relevant across the entire lifespan, participants are encouraged to think about these matters as early as possible, as opposed to doing so only on their deathbeds. Encouragingly, feedback on these sessions has been very positive. Participants are willing to share their views, and there are clear signals that many of them have already reflected on end-of-life issues beforehand, despite not necessarily knowing how to express and document their thoughts (Fig. 4.13). On this account, the sessions precisely serve an empowering role by facilitating the participants to initiate and get involved in an advance care plan on their own. Indeed, a significant portion of participants has taken the initiative to launch the communication process, or even sign the relevant documents, after attending the sessions.

Fig. 4.13 Outcome evaluation of ACP family sessions (*N*=87)

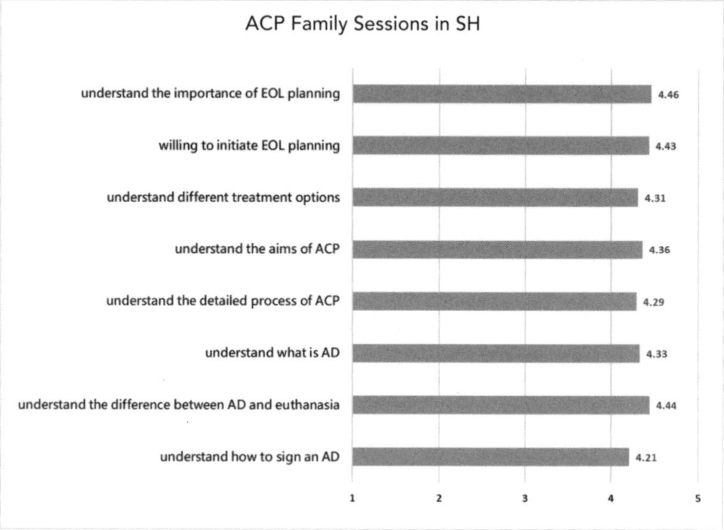

ACP Family Sessions in SH

understand the importance of EOL planning	4.46
willing to initiate EOL planning	4.43
understand different treatment options	4.31
understand the aims of ACP	4.36
understand the detailed process of ACP	4.29
understand what is AD	4.33
understand the difference between AD and euthanasia	4.44
understand how to sign an AD	4.21

Besides the workshops on advance care planning, the Institute has also conducted other educational programmes to raise public knowledge and awareness of end-of-life issues in general (Fig. 4.14). For instance, the Institute organised the Dying Matters Awareness Event in 2020, which was a series of large-scale educational activities and promotional campaigns aiming to engage the general public in active and open discussions about end-of-life issues. There were various components in the event, including, in particular, a territory-wide drawing competition, a mini concert, and the filming of a micro-movie. Again, the general public is not considered passive recipients of knowledge but is transformed into an active participator in the advance care planning process. Enthusiastic feedback from the public is shown by the quantitative evaluation results as documented in a summary report. For instance, when participants were asked to rate the effects on different aspects of the public education programmes (the score is from 1 to 5, with 5 representing highest agreement), it is found that the participants had increased their knowledge of end-of-life planning (mean score = 4.33/5), became more willing to discuss and plan for end-of-life issues (mean score = 4.21/5), and would seek more information on end-of-life issues in the future (mean score = 4.31/5). It can be seen that the educational activities have not only instilled knowledge but have also created attitudinal and behavioural changes among the general public, thereby generating an empowering effect on society and achieving a sustainable impact (CUHKIOA, 2016a, 2016b, 2016c, 2016d, 2016e, 2017a, 2017b, 2017c, 2017d, 2018a, 2018b, 2018c, 2018d, 2018e, 2018f, 2018g, 2019a, 2019b, 2019c, 2020a, 2020b, 2020c, 2020d, 2020e, 2021a, 2021b, 2021c, 2021d, 2022a).

Dying Matters Awareness Event organised by the Institute of Ageing

A series of educational activities and promotional campaigns in 2020:

- Online talks (1,766 participants)
- Drawing competition (260 entries)
- MTR Art Community Gallery
- Mini concert
- Micro-movie + celebrity interview
- Social media: 19,535 views (as at 10 Jan 2023) on Facebook page and 332,963 views (as at 10 Jan 2023) on YouTube channel

An example of this is the drawing competition, in which participants—through the titles and descriptions of their drawings—reflected their thoughts and expressions of the wish to make fulfilled end-of-life care plans (Fig. 4.15).

Fig. 4.14 Publications of the ACP. Educational Materials for the general public: *At Ease Kit* (《安心包》), *ACP Handbook* (《晚晴照顧手冊》), *Good Death Please* (《吾該好死》). Number of copies distributed: 34,250 (as at 10 Jan 2023)

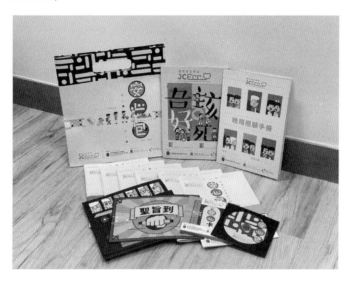

Fig. 4.15a: Winner of the drawing competition in the general public category. Title: 'The Road of Life'

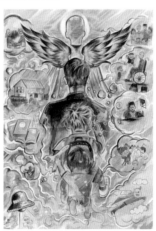

Fig. 4.15b: Winner of the drawing competition in the tertiary students' category. Title: 'The most meaningful end of life'

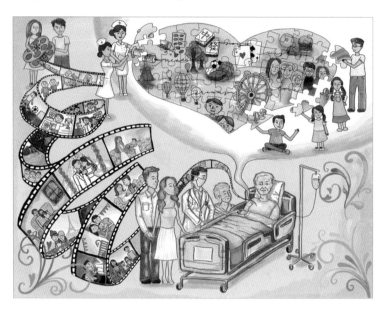

Fig. 4.15c: Winner of the drawing competition in the older people category. Title: 'A Life of No Regrets'

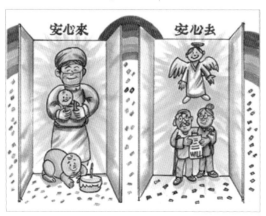

Useful Links of the EOLC Project

- Homepage: https://www.ioa.cuhk.edu.hk/end-of-life-care/
- Videos: https://www.ioa.cuhk.edu.hk/end-of-life-care/resources/#resources-button
- Publications: https://www.ioa.cuhk.edu.hk/end-of-life-care/resources/for-general-public-leaflet/
- Dying Matters Awareness Event: https://www.ioa.cuhk.edu.hk/end-of-life-care/dying-matters-awareness-event/
- Facebook page: https://www.facebook.com/LiveFreeDieWell.IOA/
- YouTube Channel: https://www.youtube.com/channel/UC9HDwKtdsljk-dyZdpcdlRZw

---

Changing Social Mindset

In parallel with the empowerment of individuals to achiever healthy ageing, similar processes need to take place for society as a whole. There is a need to remove the predominantly negative image of ageing as people on the fringe of society without a voice, who are passive recipients of care, dependent, poor and ignorant. A comparison between the situation in Hong Kong and the US with its American Association of Retired Persons (www.aarp.org), the largest organisation in the US—with about 38 million members dedicated to empowering Americans 50 and older to choose how they live as they age—illustrates how far societal opinions and the mindset in Hong Kong need to change. Importantly, health and social care professionals have a crucial role in not persevering with the narrative that ageing equates with chronic disease and hence prevention should focus on screening and management of non-communicable diseases—thus neglecting geriatric syndromes that have a similar impact on healthcare expenditures in addition to the quality of life of older adults. Declining rates of non-communicable diseases should not be used as the sole indicator of healthy ageing.

In the current United Nations Decade of Healthy Ageing, the World Health Organization's Healthy Ageing Report has been adopted, which promotes integrated care for older persons as a response to population ageing in high, middle, and low-income countries. Healthy ageing incorporates a life course approach and social justice.

Institutions could lead by adopting practices that promote healthy ageing. Recently, the concept of anchor institutions has been promoted in overseas studies. These institutions, such as hospitals and universities, usually have a significant stake in their local area, and have sizeable resources which could support their local community's health and well-being and tackle health inequalities.

The UK is spearheading this concept with the publication of the Marmot Report for Business commissioned by Legal and General (L&G), a world-wide company that manages pension funds among other business activities. Twelve areas under the categories of employees, clients and customers, and communities are highlighted to show what companies (and organisations) can do to promote health equity (Fig. 4.16) (Marmot et al, 2022).

Ultimately, this may translate into increased productivity, reduced staff turnover, and sickness absences. This philosophy may be disseminated by L&G choosing investments in other companies that follow these principles, in the same way that Environmental, Social, and Governance (ESG) principles are disseminated. The Report calls for adding the health component

Fig. 4.16 How businesses shape health: The UCL Institute of Health Equity framework

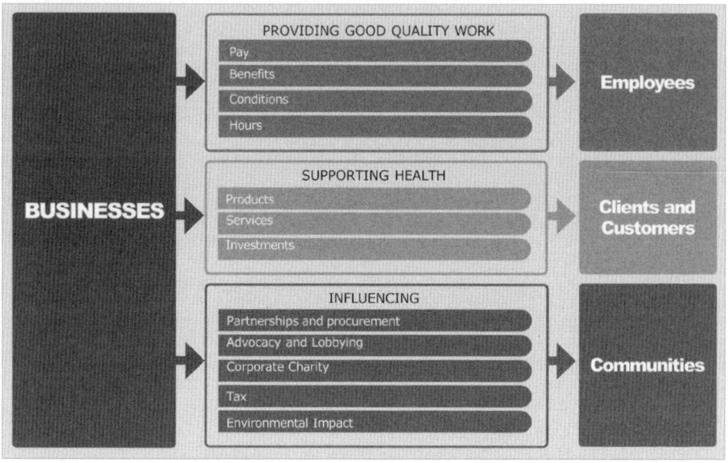

to make this ESHG. This movement is an example of the emergence of anchor institutions, which are committed to tackling the social determinants of health through changing the way staff are employed, procurement of goods and services, using their physical and environmental assets, and partnering with others. Five principles for embedding equity in anchor institution work have been proposed and piloted in the setting of National Health Service Foundation Trusts (Allen et al., 2022).

Government Policies: Advocate for a Cross-Sectoral Approach

The Hong Kong government has provided various measures in terms of allowances, as well as vouchers for health, day care and residential care (which allow choice and so perhaps indirectly drive quality improvement for service providers through market competition). However, these benefits are not widely known and the navigation complicated. Social welfare expenditure represented $81.6 billion and 18.6% of recurrent government expenditure and 2.87% of GDP in 2019–2020 (HKSAR, 2021). Yet there are unmet needs in spite of various new initiatives such as dementia day care centres. The use of vouchers of varying degrees of government subvention illustrate the principle of proportionate universalism in mitigating the impact of income inequalities.

Interviews of relatives of attendees at a dementia day care centre in a public housing estate showed five main themes: carer burden that is hardly bearable in the absence of such services; difficulties in choosing/accessing such services; the benefits of day care service; the importance of government financial support in facilitating equitable care; and the role of non-governmental organisations and social workers in bridging the information gap (Chan et al., 2022). Development of integrated systems in primary care is being promoted in many countries. Many non-governmental organisations have started to take on elements of primary care screening followed by referrals to District Health Centres or organizing group intervention programmes, such as for frailty (Woo, 2022b).

Since frailty increases the utilisation of hospital services and risk of dependency, screening for frailty and intervention programmes are just as important as the focus on hypertension and diabetes. The prevalence of frailty and pre-frailty combined is as high as hypertension, yet this aspect of ageing has been neglected by policy makers and ignored as being important for public health, in spite of the fact that it has been recognised as a public health problem (BGS; Cesari et al., 2016). The current public health narrative is still only chronic disease focused, on hypertension and diabetes. The government has strategies and action plans to prevent and control non-communicable diseases, but nothing similar is found to tackle frailty of older people.

Nevertheless, in recent years a network of district based local health centres—District Health Centres—has been established, working closely with local non-governmental organisations as well as family practitioners, thus strengthening the community and services domain of the Age-friendly Cities movement. Such centres have the potential to address the challenges of population ageing by addressing both chronic diseases as well as geriatric syndromes such as frailty, sarcopenia, and memory impairment.

There is an urgent need for a cross-sectoral approach in government policies for social welfare and health, in response to pandemics and disasters.

NGOs and Potential Anchor Institutions: The Role of Civil Society in Health Care

Similar to the principles of the ICOPE model proposed by the WHO, in Hong Kong a pilot E-health project initiated by the Hong Kong Jockey Club Charities Trust, in collaboration with 100 community NGO centres and the Chinese University of Hong Kong, has been evolving since 2016. The project was designed to apply digital technologies to empower older people in health management and promote primary care services in the context of community centres that are responsive to their needs. In essence, deficits in the domains of intrinsic capacity are detected using automated means (Fig. 4.17), followed by an action pathway. This platform allows regular follow-up assessments to monitor changes and evaluate the effectiveness of any intervention programmes. Screening results show that there is a high prevalence of impairments in intrinsic capacity domains, with 85% with one or more impairments and 27% with three or more impairments (Yu et al., 2022). The number of impaired domains predicted the incidence of polypharmacy (simultaneous use of multiple medicines), incontinence, poor/fair self-rated health, and instrumental activities of daily living after three years of follow-up. Intervention programmes have been designed to be carried out by centre staff. The latter agreed that the ICOPE principles could be implemented in the community setting, and further development of these programmes is important in contributing to the community and services of individual districts, forming the bottom layer in a step care approach to primary care of older adults. With increased manpower, this approach could form one of the key pillars of primary care, potentially linking up with District Health Centres and local family doctors.

Fig. 4.17 Healthcare needs of participants in the pilot E-health project

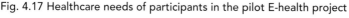
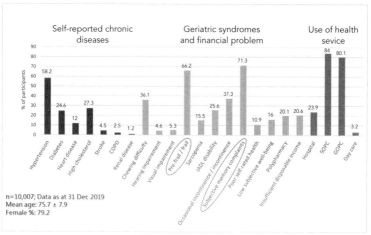

A Digital Questionnaire (Well-being Survey) for Screening of Health Status

Objective of the digital questionnaire:
To promote elderly centres as the first point of contact for detecting and addressing the health and social needs of older people

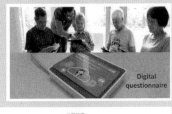

Digital questionnaire

Design of the questionnaire covers various domains such as:

- Chronic diseases
- Cognitive function
- Frailty
- Sarcopenia
- Oral health & sensory
- Psychological well-being
- Incontinence
- Self-rated health
- Medications
- Instrumental Activities of Daily Living (IADL)

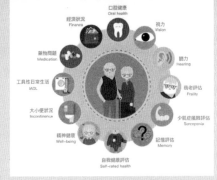

An earlier demonstration project in a public housing estate adopting similar principles of integrated care was started in 2009 and run as a self-financing model (Woo et al., 2021). This is a new model providing one-stop services, including screening for healthy ageing indicators and common chronic diseases such as hypertension and diabetes, programmes targeting domains with deficits, and rehabilitation and day care for dependent older adults. The primary care section includes a Traditional Chinese Medicine clinic, optometry, nutrition and nurse counselling. Group exercise programmes, talks, and self-measurement of blood pressure and body mass index are encouraged. There is also an exercise circuit

Fig. 4.18 Profile of the cases

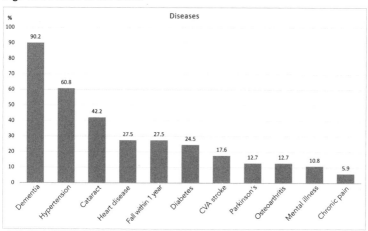

with Smart Fit equipment that provides objective measures of strength of difference muscle groups, directed by a physical trainer (https://jcch.org.hk/phc_health_promo/#smart). The day care section aims to optimize physical and cognitive function of dependent older adults and provide training and support to their carers. Fig 4.18 provides illustrations of some of the cases and the impact of such services.

Care provided by the centres covers many domains, as shown on p. 72.

One patient with stroke attended a day care centre. He improved in mood and also in function in this setting. However, he was sent to a residential care home because of family disagreements about his care plan. While at the care home, he continued to attend the centre. He was very unhappy at the care home and his mobility also deteriorated. After several discussions with centre staff, they eventually agreed to look after him at home again. One

Service Needs of Cases

Physical domain: Diagnosis of urinary tract infection; adjustment of hypertensive medication after hypotensive episode

Psychological domain: Post-bereavement depression support; resolving marital disharmony

Functional status: Post-hip fracture rehabilitation

Nutritional domain: Malnutrition reversed by hub services

Social domain: Carer support/respite care/alternative to residential care

Advance care planning: Choice of artificial feeding in late-stage dementia

80-year-old woman was in hospital for many weeks with various complications after surgery. On discharge, she attended the centre for mobilization and day care. Her medical prognosis was not good. A space-occupying lesion was found in her brain and neurosurgeons recommended hospital admission for procedures. She adamantly refused and stated that she would never enter hospital again even if she died. Centre staff discussed end-of-life care wishes of the patient and her family, and helped with advance care planning, including choice of life-sustaining treatments such as artificial feeding, mechanical ventilation, and cardio-pulmonary resuscitation.

Comments from Carers about Day Care Centre

- Helps with difficulties of caregiving
- Place for health maintenance activities
- Provision of skilled care
- Relieves carer stress and improves family relationships
- Government subsidy is very important in enabling them to use this service

Impacts of Day Care Centre
- Addresses unmet needs
- Addresses health inequalities by tackling social as well as behavioural determinants for prevention of age-related decline and promoting health span
- Government day care vouchers with value depending on income is a key feature of mitigating health inequalities using this service model
- Allows scaling up of social enterprises and further development of integrated care.

A key feature of these community initiatives is identifying the gaps in terms of unmet needs, from the older person and/or their carer's perspectives. In the absence of government funding, there is the flexibility to design and modify programmes with evaluation, to arrive at a model that is sustainable on a self-funded basis with support from philanthropic organisations. Potential users effectively help shape the development of such services. Service design requires an understanding of what motivates older people to change their lifestyle in order to retard the ageing process; what ensures the incorporation of behavioural change into their daily life; and the affordability of such programmes. Inclusion of elements of co-creation will be important, in contrast to the predominantly paternalistic exchange between the medical sector and patients. As an accompaniment, an important part of evaluation of effectiveness would be patient-related outcome measures. These measures are framed differently to the standard health research tools or outcomes that can be measured objectively. Nevertheless, they are just as important. For example, in the Cadenza Hub frailty prevention programme mentioned above that seeks to maintain/improve physical and cognitive function, a focus group discussion regarding why they participated on a regular basis for many years showed that a most commonly expressed reason is that 'they feel better'. Although evaluation of the programme did reveal improvement in frailty status as well as cognitive function that is statistically significant, this fact will not be as important as the 'feeling better' factor in adoption of this programme into their regular lifestyle (Yu et al., 2021; Yu, So, et al., 2020; Yu, Tong, Ho, et al., 2020).

These new service models involve co-payment by the user as well as government subsidies, using the existing mechanisms of health, day care and residential care vouchers. They also explore harnessing technological innovations for healthy ageing. In future, health technology assessments should be carried out to determine the economic and social benefits of such service models.

The Age-friendly Cities movement also promotes changes in the social and physical environments in which people grow old, and is one of the four areas of action of the UN Decade of Healthy Ageing 2020–2030. Age-friendly communities directly address the importance of creating an age-friendly environment to foster active and healthy ageing. Building age-friendly environments is vital to maintaining the intrinsic capacity of older people, as well as helping their autonomy, dignity and well-being. In Hong Kong, the success of its preventive health services enables the population to have the longest life expectancy at birth in the world, surpassing that of Japan. Its compactness and contrasting urban and open spaces possess many advantages for ageing people to live in.

The concept of the influence of the physical and social environmental factors as determinants of health, in addition to the role of personal social determinants of health such as lifestyle and socioeconomic characteristics, began to be promoted in the early 2000s in a collection of essays from a transdisciplinary perspective (Woo, 2013). A detailed description to explore the age-friendliness of Hong Kong covering opportunities, initiatives and challenges may be found elsewhere (Philips et al., 2019). These two bodies of work, inspired by the World Health Organization's Age-friendly Cities philosophy, together with the AFC initiative from the Hong Kong Council for Social Service representing the territories' non-governmental organisations providing community services for older adults, laid the foundation for a major territory-wide AFC initiative led by the Hong Kong Jockey Club Charities Trust in collaboration with academia, non-governmental organizations, district councils (DCs), and businesses in 2016. The age-friendliness of each district was assessed based on the eight AFC domains, the results of which guided the drawing up of three-year action plans and district-based programmes in consultation with district councils and district stakeholders. Leveraging on the Trust's strong network, a multi-sectoral collaboration was formed, consisting of 18 district councils, corresponding District Offices and various government departments; a partnership with four gerontological research institutes to engage professional sectors and the broader community; active involvement of more than 70 non-governmental organisations in building up an age-friendly momentum; and participation of over 180 companies and/or organisations from the business and public sectors in the form of the Jockey Club Age-friendly City Partnership Scheme. The four research institutes worked together to carry out baseline and final assessments of the age-friendliness of all 18 districts using a mixed methods approach;

at the same time, the local indicators of age-friendliness were benchmarked with international data. The ultimate objective of these initiatives is to insert the concept of age-friendliness into all facets of society, such that the ultimate sustainability of the project will hopefully be reflected in the improvement and continuing development in all eight domains.

To understand the needs of older people in the local community and therefore identify areas of improvement for future action and change, the Jockey Club Age-friendly City (JCAFC) Project conducted a baseline assessment study, comprising quantitative and qualitative methods, to assess the level of age-friendliness of 8 AFC domains in 18 districts of Hong Kong from 2015 to 2017. Overall, more than 9,700 respondents completed the survey questionnaire and over 700 participants joined the focus group interviews (91 focus groups in total) in 18 districts. Among the eight domains, social participation (4.29 out of 6) and transportation (4.27 out of 6) scored the highest, whereas civic participation and employment (3.87 out of 6), housing (3.71 out of 6) and community support and health services (3.67 out of 6) scored the lowest (Table 4.1). The scores of domains for each district can be found at the webpage https://www.jcafc.hk/en/Project-Components/Comprehensive-Support-Scheme-For-Districts/Baseline-Assessment-And-Action-Plans.html. The results of the baseline assessment provided the evidence for the JCAFC Project to engage with the stakeholders of local districts (e.g., DCs/District Officers, and NGOs) to discuss and develop district-tailored action plans that addressed the lower-scoring AFC domains, and proposed appropriate strategies and action steps on improving the age-friendliness in 18 districts.

Table 4.1 Scores of AFC domains at the baseline assessment in 18 districts

Age-friendly City Domains	Mean Scores
Social participation	4.29
Transportation	4.27
Respect and social inclusion	4.10
Communication and information	4.06
Outdoor spaces and buildings	4.04
Civic participation and employment	3.87
Housing	3.71
Community support and health services	3.67

Note: Survey participants were asked to rate the items on a 6-point Likert scale, ranging from 1 (strongly disagree) to 6 (strongly agree) to indicate the extent to which they perceive age-friendly features in the district they live. The higher the score, the higher the perceived level of age-friendliness on the item(s) being measured.

The Institute of Ageing also developed a local AgeWatch Index for Hong Kong to assess elderly well-being in a comprehensive manner with locally significant indicators annually, starting in 2014, for six consecutive years. Based on 13 indicators in four domains (i.e., income security, health status, capability, and enabling environment) proposed in the Global AgeWatch Index, Hong Kong was ranked 24th among 97 countries and territories in 2014. In terms of the domains, Hong Kong performed well in enabling environment (rank 4th) and health status (rank 9th), average in capability (rank 33rd), but poor in income security (rank 75th) (Fig. 4.19). In 2016, the AgeWatch Index was further expanded to the Hong Kong Elder Quality of Life Index (HKEQOL Index). The HKEQOL Index includes tailor-made indicators for Hong Kong about the AFC concept proposed by the World Health Organization and makes reference to the Global AgeWatch Index, using 22 indicators in the same four core domains. It enables trend analysis of the social and economic well-being of older people annually,

Fig. 4.19 AgeWatch Index rankings for Hong Kong, 2014

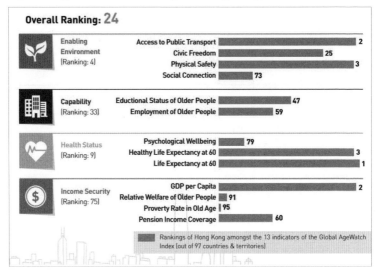

as well as monitoring and evaluating local age-friendly initiatives (CUHKIOA 2018g, 2020c, 2020d, 2020e).

The above initiatives describe what can be done in Hong Kong in the area of age-friendly environments, providing a beginning to action on one of the four areas of the UN Decade of Healthy Ageing. It is also a good example of what philanthropy, academia, and non-governmental organisations can achieve in addressing societal challenges that require a cross-sectoral and cross-disciplinary approach.

By taking charge of our own ageing, we will be able to shape how Hong Kong society can deal with the implications of an ageing population. As shown in the preceding paragraphs, using the perspective of older people themselves, we should continue to collect evidence of what the needs are, contribute to designing and supporting pilot models of services in the community, provide input to businesses, housing design and senior living arrangements, and urban planning of the neighbourhood environment. It has been estimated that in 2020, consumer spending by those aged 50+ represented 50% of the total, contributed 34% to GDP, and created 1 billion jobs. By 2050 these figures are estimated to be 59%, 39% and 1.5 billion (Accius et al, 2022).

Ageing in place cannot happen without factors that enable healthy ageing and that take account of the continuity of ageing itself and accompanied changes. Housing models that adopt a cross-sectional approach to a sector of the life course may not be the answer. Architects and designers need to understand age-related changes from an older person's perspective. For example, with age, there is increased prevalence of cataracts. Through the eyes of someone with cataracts, furniture can be hard to see in rooms decorated in a light cream colour scheme, but may be seen more clearly in rooms with sharp contrasts such as black and white. Depth perception, colour contrast and dark adaptation may also be impaired. Steps may be missed if they are entirely black and glossy, or entirely creamy. In recent years, architects, designers, and property companies have started to seek the opinions of older adults in their projects.

Chapter Five

WHAT ARE OTHER COUNTRIES DOING?

Study tours to other countries are very popular among government officials and staff of NGOs. For tours on ageing and related issues such as senior living and use of gerontechnology, Japan, Scandinavian countries and the Netherlands are some of the destinations. Singapore, nearer to those of us living in Hong Kong, has a Ministry of Health Transformation to undertake the transformation of health systems to be patient-centred, data driven and digitally enabled, and to better empower health, prevent disease, and provide excellent value-based care. The strategy is to create health precincts-designed geographical areas that are conducive to healthy behaviours, through co-creation of age-friendly neighbourhoods that take into account socio-environmental determinants of behaviour. Paul Ong, the Chief Strategy Officer of the Tsao Foundation, summarizes the approach to the 100-year life realistically: to enable a meaningful life without full health, and empowering the 'consumer' rather than the 'patient'.

●　　●　　●

Integrated Care as a Feature of Universal Health Coverage

As part of the UN Decade of Healthy Ageing, the World Health Organization continues to promote the core areas for healthy ageing world-wide. Notably it promotes a model of universal health coverage that consists of integrated health and social care to maximize intrinsic capacity and functional ability as part of primary care responses to older people's needs. The long-term impact of the programme is expected to improve healthy life expectancy, well-being, reduce care dependency, cause and quality of death. The meeting of the WHO Clinical Consortium for Health Ageing (CCHA) in November 2022 illustrates what various countries are doing. An ICOPE screening app has already been developed in eight different languages, available for download free of charge. Initiatives range from training of ICOPE assessments and validation of the intrinsic capacity assessment tools, to pilots of using the ICOPE screening in the community. France is spearheading the incorporation of the ICOPE programme in clinical practice in the primary care setting. The primary objective is to test the feasibility of incorporating the ICOPE programme into existing primary care structures, with the aid of technology. Baseline screening of 10,903 older people was carried out, with 9.3% then progressing to in-depth assessments, followed by care plans, mainly in the areas relating to locomotion, vitality and cognition (Tavassoli et al., 2022).

An ICOPE manual has been produced for training in Southeast Asian countries by the WHO Regional Office for South-East Asia. In China, a large-scale training programme for home care service workers is being rolled out, with government support. By 2050, the percentage of people aged 65 and above in China is projected to be 47% of the total population, and the growth of dependent older adults projected to reach 96 million. The consequence of population ageing has been accorded high importance by the Chinese government and included as a national strategy in the 14th Five-Year Plan. Among the 20 major indicators, 7 are related to people's well-being. As a matter of urgency, the WHO ICOPE China Pilot for feasibility was carried out starting in September 2020 in the Chaoyang District of Beijing, for 2,200 older adults. The pilot consisted of screening, followed by an intervention care plan and holistic care cycle, with evaluation. Using automated methods, screening was self-administered, and intervention provided online or offline. Evaluation included a comparison control group. The ICOPE concept was promoted widely through local networks. Intrinsic capacity measurements were followed up for a six-month period in a selected sub-sample. This model is being rolled out to 13 cities in China, to include all the elements described above. Data to be collected for evaluation include change in function and health status, lifestyle and well-being changes, changes in health resource utilisation and service satisfaction. For service providers, satisfaction towards programme implementation and work satisfaction will be assessed, together with caregiver burden indicators for family members. Direct and indirect costs for this model of care will also be estimated. Other countries in Europe, Japan, and Latin America are actively exploring the feasibility of this integrated model of care for older people.

In China, the concept of integration of medical and elderly care has been raised and developed since 2015. Amongst various modes of integration are setting up medical facilities in elderly care facilities (or vice versa) and signing collaboration agreements between elderly care and medical facilities for better resources sharing and service provision. A speech by an official in China in May 2023 revealed that by the end of 2022, 84,000 connected pairs of elderly care and medical facilities have signed collaboration agreements while 6,986 institutions have integrated the two types of services offering 1,850,000 beds.

Government-Run Pensions and Insurance Schemes

Many Asian countries such as China, Japan, Korea, and Singapore have in place pension, health insurance and long-term care insurance schemes that are funded by contributions by the working population and the government. In China, for example, its long-term care insurance system, which focuses on guaranteeing the basic life care and medical care of severely disabled persons, has been implemented in 49 cities covering 170 million people. Use of services usually involves some co-payment. A co-payment model based on insurance will likely be more sustainable compared with a predominantly taxation based or out-of-pocket models.

Businesses Contribute to Healthy Ageing

As discussed in Chapter Four, the role of the business sector in creating a conducive work environment and the impact that has on employees' health has been in the spotlight in recent years. Likewise, any negative effects on employees' health due to their work environment not being conducive can carry on into their retirement and continue to affect their health. The same is true for organisations, which have the same responsibility to create an environment that supports the health of the communities in different ways.

In the UK, the Legal and General Insurance Group commissioned the University College London Institute of Health Equity to produce a report that sets out the principles for how businesses and organisations in general may shape health. The report states that they did this by providing good quality work on the part of employees built on pay, benefits, conditions and working hours; by supporting health in terms of products, services and investments for their clients and customers; and benefiting wider communities such as providing housing and facilities by influencing partnerships and procurements, advocacy and lobbying, corporate charity, tax, and environmental impact (Marmot et al., 2022).

Housing and Ageing in Place

Various models have been adopted by other countries such as Australia, Singapore, the UK, Norway, and the US to enable older people to continue to live in communities rather than live in residential care. These include leisure orientated residential communities such as retirement villages, independent living housing arrangements with some housing maintenance support, and various forms of continuing care retirement communities (Ko et al., 2021). For instance, Australia's government addresses the diverse needs of older people by expanding dwelling options available in the community to promote ageing in place. The demand by older people for smaller sized housing with age-friendly designs is met through assistance on home modification, delivering good quality new housing, and funding through community support programmes, providing older people with different level of independence. In the UK, the government has introduced progressive building regulations to foster an elderly-friendly environment for older people in mainstream housing design, with three tiers of standards: visitable dwellings, accessible and adaptable dwellings, and wheelchair-user dwellings. Although the latter two standards have no binding effect, it serves as a benchmark for others to follow and help improve the community by ensuring accessibility, flexibility, adaptability and inclusivity in its built environment. In the US, ensuring affordability to a safe and decent living based on the preference of older people is the key to address the concerns of older people. Reverse mortgage programmes allow elders to use part of their asset wealth for immediate use without compromising their right to live in their homes. Some states such as New York State have created Naturally Occurring Retirement Communities (NORCs) to facilitate older people ageing in place. NORCs are available for a group of 250 older residents in a building, or 500 older residents in a community, where at least 40% of the units have an occupant who is an older adult, and a majority of the older adults are low to medium income. Social and healthcare resources are available in NORCs at affordable prices through matching funds from the government. Residents can also gain access to resources such as transport assistance and home adaption services.

Various modes of living are supported in these settings, including independent living, assisted living, senior co-living, and multi-generational co-living. Similarly, various types of support services are available elsewhere, depending on the mode of funding. For example, in Singapore, the Housing and Development Board, working together with the Ministry of National Development and the Ministry of Health, is expanding various housing options for older people. Following the largely successful development known as Kampung Admiralty, which brings together senior-friendly residences at a very accessible site with a mix of public facilities such as medical centres and a community garden under one roof, the joint effort further contributes to the concept of Community Care Apartments (CCA) (Figs. 5.1–5.2).

Residents sign a long contract which covers the flat price and basic care services, such as 24-hour emergency monitoring and basic health checks. The complex also features communal spaces on every floor to promote social interaction, shared activities and community participation. Onsite staff will also liaise with relevant service providers as optional services to meet health and other needs, as well as facilitate a healthy lifestyle. Lately, CCA has stated that it intends to provide bigger flat sizes (e.g., three- and four-room flats) to encourage intergenerational bonding. This integrated and holistic design has become a standard approach in the planning of all new public housing in Singapore.

Fig. 5.1 Elderly-friendly design and facilities in Singapore's Community Care Apartments

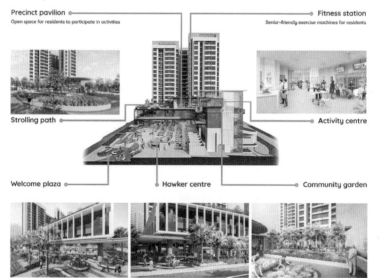

Precinct pavilion
Open space for residents to participate in activities

Fitness station
Senior-friendly exercise machines for residents

Strolling path

Activity centre

Welcome plaza

Hawker centre

Community garden

Credit: Housing & Development Board & Ministry of Health (Government of Singapore)
Source: https://www.hdb.gov.sg/about-us/news-and-publications/press-releases/10122020-Singapores-First-Assisted-Living-Flats-to-be-Launched-in-February-2021.

Hong Kong may examine and adopt some of these models, but efforts should be made to fit local needs and guard against purchasing and installation of products and copying models without adaptation.

Fig. 5.2 A rooftop community park overlooked by the flats promotes healthy living for the residents in Kampung Admiralty, Singapore

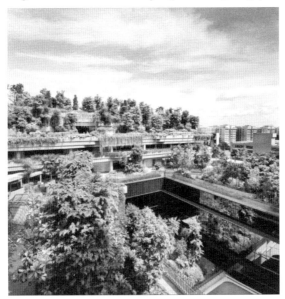

Credit: Patrick Bingham-Hall and WOHA.
Source: https://woha.net/project/kampung-admiralty/.

CONCLUSION

Demographic changes in Hong Kong raise many societal challenges, similar to Western countries such as the UK and the US, where increasing total life expectancy at birth seem to have stalled or decreased, as a result of socioeconomic inequalities, lifestyle factors, and the COVID-19 pandemic. Currently in the UK, one-fifth of the lifespan is spent in poor health, and there is a 20-year healthy life expectancy between rich and poor, which is following a widening trend. If we are concerned about healthy ageing, we need regularly collected data to monitor the trend for healthy life expectancy and to formulate health and social care policies to ensure that increase in total life expectancy is not accompanied by a static or falling healthy life expectancy, resulting in the rapidly increased burden of chronic disease and dependencies. Hong Kong should not be satisfied that increasing life expectancy at birth represents the success of health and social care systems, but should collect relevant data regarding healthy life expectancy and prepare for the future using a cross-sectoral approach as proposed by the Quantum Healthy Longevity blueprint (Woods et al., 2022). The latter adopts a societal approach, covering all the cumulative factors that contribute to disease and the accelerated ageing process (lifestyle, psychological, physical and social environment), use of technologies, promoting brain health, intergenerational and digital engagement, health equity and compassion as a core societal value. An index based on these concepts is being developed, so that health may be added to the Environmental, Social, and Governance framework criteria that is being widely adopted by various companies and organisations, to create an ESHG framework. This approach involves the whole of society and is not just the responsibility of health service providers. We all need to be a part of this movement to maximize our healthy ageing potential. We need to understand that achieving healthy ageing goes beyond prevention of non-communicable diseases, to tackling (and retarding) the ageing process itself. The latter can only be achieved by collaborative networks in ageing biology and clinical translation.

The quest for achieving healthy ageing should include considerations of social determinants using a life course approach. Social determinants should be integrated into policies in addition to health and social welfare, using the principle of universal proportionalism, whereby those most in need receive proportionately more support, as exemplified by the Dementia Day Care model (Chan et al., 2022).

Much work needs to be done to achieve healthy ageing as proposed by the UN Decade of Healthy Ageing, together with suggested guidelines for countries to formulate policies. Although Hong Kong is not a country but a special administrative region of

China, it has its own health and social welfare policies. Currently, it has an ageing population with the longest life expectancy at birth, and there is a need to formulate holistic policies towards healthy ageing. Policies need to be shaped by older people themselves if they are to be truly client centred rather than service provider centred. To achieve this goal, we need to promote a change in societal mindsets; adopt a cross-sectoral approach; tackle long term care; screen for age-related syndromes other than non-communicable diseases, followed by intervention programmes. It is encouraging that various projects in recent years have adopted this approach, supported by the Jockey Club Charities Trust. For example, the Jockey Club Design Institute for Social Innovation (JCDISI) emphasizes co-creation and innovation in design, covering the eight domains of the World Health Organization's Age-friendly Cities concept (CUHKIOA, 2016a, 2016b, 2018b, 2018c, 2018d); the various Jockey Club Trust initiated projects mentioned in the previous chapters (AFC; E-health; E-tools; End-of-Life Care; and the Cadenza Hub model).

The concept of ageing in place has attracted housing providers to develop models based on focus group data on what older people would like to see. Also following the principles of the Marmot Report for businesses, one property company headquartered in Hong Kong has pioneered the possibility of a four-and-a-half day work week with a view to addressing the work-life balance and improve job satisfaction. It is possible that such strategies not only do not reduce work output, but have the potential to increase productivity and reduce sickness absences. Ultimately, these changes should start with ourselves, by taking charge of our own ageing and participating in the co-creation of social enterprises that contribute to healthy ageing, as well as influencing government policies.

To sum up, we need to think in terms of a 100-year life, where healthy ageing does not mean focusing on the absence of diseases, but on extension of the health span taking into account the social determinants of healthy ageing. We need to think about how and where we work and live, in addition to financial management in response to the aim of extending health span. We need to take charge of our own ageing by changing our mindset to avoid self-directed ageism, as well as proactively contributing to co-creation of a physical and social environment that enables healthy ageing.

REFERENCES

Accius, J., Ladner, J., & Alexander, S. (2022). *The global longevity economy® outlook: People age 50 and older are making unprecedented economic contributions and creating opportunity for every generation.* Washington, DC: AARP Thought Leadership, November 2022. https://doi.org/10.26419/int.00052.001

Allen, M., Marmot, M., & Allwood, D. (2022). Taking one step further: Five equity principles for hospitals to increase their value as anchor institutions. *Future Healthcare Journal, 9*(3), 216– 221. https://pubmed.ncbi.nlm.nih.gov/36561807/

Bloom, D. E. (2022). Healthy ageing for a healthy economy. WHO Clinical Consortium on Healthy Ageing, Geneva.

British Geriatrics Society (BGS). *Fit for Frailty, Part 1.* https://www.bgs.org.uk/sites/default/files/content/resources/files/2018-05-14/fff2_short_0.pdf

Cesari, M., Prince, M., Thiyagarajan, J. A., De Carvalho, I. A., Bernabei, R., Chan, P., Gutierrez-Robledo, L. M., Michel, J. P., Morley, J. E., Ong, P., Rodriguez Manas, L., Sinclair, A., Won, C. W., Beard, J.,

& Vellas, B. (2016). Frailty: An emerging public health priority. *Journal of the American Medical Directors Association*, *17*(3), 188–192. https://doi.org/10.1016/j.jamda.2015.12.016

Chan, P. H., McGhee, S. M., & Woo, J. (2013). Population aging: Impact of common chronic diseases on health and social services. In J. Woo (Ed.), *Aging in Hong Kong: A comparative perspective* (pp. 115–156). Springer.

Chan, S. M., Chung, G. K., Kwan, M. H., & Woo, J. (2022). Mitigating inequalities in community care needs of older adults with dementia: A qualitative case study of an integrated model of community care operated under the proportionate universalism principle. *BMC Primary Care*, *23*(1), 244. https://doi.org/10.1186/s12875-022-01855-z

Chau, A. & Lee, R. (2022, September 30). More must be done to end inequalities Hong Kong's elderly women face. *South China Morning Post*. https://www.scmp.com/comment/letters/article/3194094/more-must-be-done-end-inequalities-hong-kongs-elderly-women-face

Cheung, J. T. K., Yu, R., Wu, Z., Wong, S. Y. S., & Woo, J. (2018). Geriatric syndromes, multimorbidity, and disability overlap and increase healthcare use among older Chinese. *BMC Geriatrics*, *18*(1), 147. https://doi.org/10.1186/s12877-018-0840-1

Chung, G. K., Robinson, M., Marmot, M., & Woo, J. (2022). Monitoring socioeconomic inequalities in health in Hong Kong: Insights and lessons from the UK and Australia. *The Lancet Regional Health - Western Pacific*, 31, 100636. https://doi.org/10.1016/j.lanwpc.2022.100636

Chung, R. Y., Lai, D. C. K., Hui, A. Y., Chau, P. Y., Wong, E. L., Yeoh, E. K., & Woo, J. (2021). Healthcare inequalities in emergency visits and hospitalisation at the end of life: A study of 395 019 public hospital records. *BMJ Supportive Palliative Care.* https://doi.org/10.1136/bmjspcare-2020-002800

Cox, L. S., & Faragher, R. G. A. (2022). Linking interdisciplinary and multiscale approaches to improve healthspan-a new UK model for collaborative research networks in ageing biology and clinical translation. The *Lancet Healthy Longevity, 3*(5), e318–e320. https://doi.org/10.1016/S2666-7568(22)00095-2

CUHKIHE. (2022). *Health inequalities in Hong Kong: A life course approach.* https://www.ihe.cuhk.edu.hk/wp-content/uploads/Health-Inequalities-in-Hong-Kong_A-Life-Course-Approach-Report.pdf

CUHKIOA. (2016a). *Jockey Club age-friendly city project action plan: Sha Tin.* https://www.jcafc.hk/uploads/docs/Sha_Tin_Action_Plan_Jun2017-(1).pdf.

CUHKIOA. (2016b). *Jockey Club age-friendly city project action plan: Tai Po.* https://www.jcafc.hk/uploads/docs/Tai_Po_Action_Plan_Jun2017.pdf

CUHKIOA. (2016c). *Jockey Club age-friendly city project baseline assessment report: Sha Tin.* https://www.jcafc.hk/uploads/docs/Shatin-output-new_20190719.pdf

CUHKIOA. (2016d). *Jockey Club age-friendly city project baseline assessment report: Tai Po.* https://www.jcafc.hk/uploads/docs/Tai_Po-output_new_20190719.pdf

CUHKIOA. (2016e). *Report on AgeWatch Index for Hong Kong 2014.* https://www.jcafc.hk/uploads/docs/Report-on-AgeWatch-Index-for-Hong-Kong-2014-(final).pdf

CUHKIOA. (2017a). *AgeWatch index for Hong Kong: Topical report on enabling environment.* https://www.jcafc.hk/uploads/docs/Topical-Report-on-Enabling-Environment-1.pdf

CUHKIOA. (2017b). *Jockey Club age-friendly city project baseline assessment report: Kwai Tsing.* https://www.jcafc.hk/uploads/docs/Kwai_Tsing_output-revised_20190719.pdf

CUHKIOA. (2017c). *Jockey Club age-friendly city project baseline assessment report: North.* https://www.jcafc.hk/uploads/docs/North-output-new_20190719.pdf

CUHKIOA. (2017d). *Jockey Club age-friendly City report baseline assessment report: Sai Kung.* https://www.jcafc.hk/uploads/docs/Sai_Kung-output-revised_20190719.pdf

CUHKIOA. (2018a). *AgeWatch index for Hong Kong: Topical report on health status.* https://www.jcafc.hk/uploads/docs/AgeWatch_Index_Topical_Report_on_Health_Status.pdf

CUHKIOA. (2018b). *Jockey Club age-friendly city project action plan: Kwai Tsing.* https://www.jcafc.hk/uploads/docs/Kwai_Tsing_Action_Plan_Feb2019.pdf

CUHKIOA. (2018c). *Jockey Club age-friendly city project action plan: North.* https://www.jcafc.hk/uploads/docs/North_Action_Plan_Feb2019.pdf

CUHKIOA. (2018d). *Jockey Club age-friendly city project action plan: Sai Kung.* https://www.jcafc.hk/uploads/docs/Sai_Kung_Action_Plan_Feb2019.pdf

CUHKIOA. (2018e). *Jockey Club age-friendly city project cross-district Report on baseline assessment (pilot districts).* https://www.jcafc.hk/uploads/docs/Cross_district_report_final_20180118_v4.pdf

CUHKIOA. (2018f). *Report on AgeWatch index for Hong Kong 2015.* https://www.jcafc.hk/uploads/docs/Report-on-AgeWatch-Index-for-Hong-Kong-2015.pdf

CUHKIOA. (2018g). *Report on AgeWatch index for Hong Kong 2016 and Hong Kong elder quality of life index.* https://www.jcafc.hk/uploads/docs/AgeWatch_Index_Report_for_HK_Yr2016(updated).pdf

CUHKIOA. (2019a). *Jockey Club age-friendly city project cross-district report of baseline assessment on age-friendliness (18 districts).* https://www.jcafc.hk/uploads/docs/Cross-district-report-of-baseline-assessment-on-age-friendliness-(18-districts).pdf

CUHKIOA. (2019b). *Jockey Club age-friendly city project final assessment report Tai Po.* https://www.jcafc-port.hk/wp-content/uploads/2022/06/Final-Assessment-report-Tai-Po.pdf

CUHKIOA. (2019c). *Jockey Club age-friendly city project final assessment report Sha Tin.* https://www.jcafc-port.hk/wp-content/uploads/2022/06/Final-Assessment-Report-Sha-Tin.pdf

CUHKIOA. (2020a). *AgeWatch index for Hong Kong: Topical report on capability.* https://www.jcafc.hk/uploads/docs/Topical-Report-Capability_final.pdf

CUHKIOA. (2020b). *AgeWatch index for Hong Kong: Topical report on income security* https://www.jcafc.hk/uploads/docs/Topical-Report-Income-Security_final.pdf

CUHKIOA. (2020c). *Report on Hong Kong elder quality of life index incorporating AgeWatch index for Hong Kong 2017.* https://www.jcafc.hk/uploads/docs/EQOL-2017_final.pdf

CUHKIOA. (2020d). *Report on Hong Kong elder quality of life index incorporating AgeWatch index for Hong Kong 2018.* https://www.jcafc.hk/uploads/docs/EQOL-2018_final.pdf

CUHKIOA. (2020e). *Report on Hong Kong elder quality of life Index incorporating AgeWatch index for Hong Kong 2019* https://www.jcafc.hk/uploads/docs/HKEQOL_2019_final_online(v2).pdf

CUHKIOA. (2021a). *Age-friendly city guidebook practical guidance and resources for Age-friendly city development in Hong Kong.* https://www.jcafc-port.hk/wp-content/uploads/2021/12/P171_Age-friendly-City-Guidebook.pdf

CUHKIOA. (2021b). *Jockey Club age-friendly city project final assessment report: Kwai Tsing.* https://www.jcafc-port.hk/wp-content/uploads/2022/12/JCAFC_Final-Assessment-Report_Kwai-Tsing_20211025.pdf

CUHKIOA. (2021c). *Jockey Club age-friendly city project final assessment report: North.* https://www.jcafc-port.hk/wp-content/uploads/2022/12/JCAFC_Final-Assessment-Report_North_20211026.pdf

CUHKIOA. (2021d). *Jockey Club age-friendly city project final assessment report: Sai Kung.* https://www.jcafc-port.hk/wp-content/uploads/2022/12/Final-Assessment-Report-Sai-Kung.pdf

CUHKIOA. (2022a). *Jockey Club age-friendly city project evaluation report.* https://www.jcafc-port.hk/wp-content/uploads/2022/05/JCAFC-Project-Evaluation-Report_final-for-web-uploading.pdf

CUHKIOA. (2022b). *Thematic report series on the concept of an age-friendly city in Hong Kong—communication and information.* https://www.jcafc.hk/uploads/docs/Thematic-report-on-Communication-and-Information.pdf

CUHKIOA. (2022c). *Thematic report series on the concept of an age-friendly city in Hong Kong—community support and health services.* https://www.jcafc-port.hk/wp-content/uploads/2022/05/Thematic-report-on-Community-Support-and-Health- Services.pdf

CUHKIOA. (2022d). *Thematic report series on the concept of an age-friendly city in Hong Kong—outdoor spaces and buildings.* https://www.jcafc-port.hk/wp-content/uploads/2022/05/Thematic-report-on-Outdoor-Spaces-and-Buildings.pdf

CUHKIOA. (2022e). *Thematic report series on the concept of an age-friendly city in Hong Kong – Transportation.* https://www.jcafc-port.hk/wp-content/uploads/2022/05/Thematic-report-on-Transportation.pdf

CUHKIOA. (2022f).《吾該活在何方？尋覓香港長者的理想居所》。[Where shall I live? Finding ideal residence for seniors.] https://www.ioa.cuhk.edu.hk/images/ehealth/ehealth_booklet22.pdf

HKSAR, Census and Statistics Department. (2019). *Hong Kong Poverty Situation Report 2018.* https://www.statistics.gov.hk/pub/B9XX0005E2018AN18E0100.pdf

HKSAR, Census and Statistics Department. (2020). *Hong Kong poverty situation report 2019.* https://www.commissiononpoverty.gov.hk/eng/pdf/Hong_Kong_Poverty_Situation_Report_2019.pdf

HKSAR, Census and Statistics Department. (2021). *Hong Kong poverty situation report 2020.* https://www.censtatd.gov.hk/en/data/stat_report/product/B9XX0005/att/B9XX0005E2020AN20e0100.PDF

Ho, S. C., Chan, A., Woo, J., Chong, P., & Sham, A. (2009). Impact of caregiving on health and quality of life: A comparative population-based study of caregivers for elderly persons and noncaregivers. *The Journals of Gerontology Series A Biological Sciences and Medical Sciences*, 64(8), 873–879. https://doi.org/10.1093/gerona/glp034

Holt-Lunstad, J. & Perissinotto, C. (2023). Social isolation and loneliness as medical issues. *The New England Journal of Medicine,* 388(3),193–195. http://doi.org/10.1056/NEJMp2208029

Hospital Authority. (2023, September 30). *Waiting time for stable new case booking at specialist out-Patient clinics.* https://www.ha.org.hk/haho/ho/sopc/dw_wait_ls_eng.pdf

Kleinman A., Eisenberg L., & Good B. (1978). Culture, illness, and care: Clinical lessons from anthropologic and cross-cultural research. *Annals of Internal Medicine; 88*(2), 251–258.

Ko et al., (2021). Research study on the residential design guide for healthy aging in Hong Kong, unpublished report.

Marmot, M., Alexander, M., Allen, J., & Munro, A. (2022). *The business of health equity: The Marmot review for industry.* UCL Institute of Health Equity.

Mavrodaris, A., Lafortune, L., & Brayne, C. E. (2022). The future longevity: Designing a synergistic approach for healthy ageing, sustainability, and equity. *The Lancet Healthy Longevity, 3*(9), e584–e586. https://doi.org/10.1016/S2666-7568(22)00145-3

Meier, E. A., Gallegos, J. V., Thomas, L. P., Depp, C. A., Irwin, S. A., & Jeste, D. V. (2016). Defining a good death (successful dying): Literature review and a call for research and public dialogue. *The American Journal of Geriatric Psychiatry, 24*(4), 261–271. https://doi.org/10.1016/j.jagp.2016.01.135

Ng, R., Allore, H. G., Trentalange, M., Monin, J. K., & Levy, B. R. (2015). Increasing negativity of age stereotypes across 200 years: Evidence from a database of 400 million words. *PLoS One, 10*(2), e0117086. https://doi.org/10.1371/journal.pone.0117086

Ni, M. Y., Canudas-Romo, V., Shi, J., Flores, F. P., Chow, M. S. C., Yao, X. I., Ho, S. Y., Lam, T. H., Schooling, C. M., Lopez, A. D., Ezzati, M., & Leung, G. M. (2021). Understanding longevity in Hong Kong: A comparative study with long-living, high-income countries. *The Lancet Public Health, 6*(12), e919–e931. https://doi.org/10.1016/S2468-2667(21)00208-5

Philips, D. R., Woo, J., Cheung, F., Wong, M., & Chau, P. H. (2019). Exploring the age-friendliness of Hong Kong: Opportunities, initiatives and challenges in an ageing Asian city. In T. Buffel, S.

handler, & C. Phillipson (Eds.), *Age-friendly Cities and Communities: A global perspective* (pp. 119–142). Policy Press.

Stroud, L. R., Salovey, P., & Epel, E. S. (2002). Sex differences in stress responses: Social rejection versus achievement stress. *Biological Psychiatry, 52*(4), 318–327. https://doi.org/10.1016/s0006-3223(02)01333-1

Tavassoli, N., de Souto Barreto, P., Berbon, C., Mathieu, C., de Kerimel, J., Lafont, C., Takeda, C., Carrie, I., Piau, A., Jouffrey, T., Andrieu, S., Nourhashemi, F., Beard, J. R., Soto Martin, M. E., & Vellas, B. (2022). Implementation of the WHO integrated care for older people (ICOPE) programme in clinical practice: A prospective study. *The Lancet Healthy Longevity, 3*(6), e394–e404. https://doi.org/10.1016/S2666-7568(22)00097-6

The Lancet Healthy Longevity. (2022). Ageing populations: Unaffordable demography. *The Lancet Healthy Longevity, 3*(12), e804. https://doi.org/10.1016/S2666-7568(22)00272-0

Thiyagarajan, J., Mikton, C., Harwood, R. H., Gichu, M., Gaigbe-Togbe, V., Jhamba, T., Pokorna, D., Stoevska, V., Hada, R., Steffan, G. S., Liena, A., Rocard, E., & Diaz, T. (2022). The UN decade of healthy ageing: Strengthening measurement for monitoring health and wellbeing of older people. *Age Ageing, 51*(7). https://doi.org/10.1093/ageing/afac147

Wang D., Lau K. K., Yu R., Wong S. Y. S., Kwok T. T. Y., & Woo J. (2017) Neighbouring green space and mortality in community-dwelling elderly Hong Kong Chinese: A cohort study. *BMJ Open*; 7(7), e015794. https://www.ncbi.nlm.nih.gov/pubmed/28765127.

Wong, M., Yu, R., & Woo, J. (2017). Effects of perceived neighbourhood environments on self-rated health among community-dwelling older Chinese. *International Journal of Environmental Research and Public Health, 14*(6). https://doi.org/10.3390/ijerph14060614

Woo, J. (2013). *Aging in Hong Kong: A comparative perspective.* Springer.

Woo, J. (2020). The myth of filial piety as a pillar for care of older adults among Chinese populations. *Advances in Geriatric Medicine and Research, 2*(2), e200012.

Woo, J. (2021). The need for an evidence based COVID-19 pandemic response policy that incorporates risk benefit considerations, that does not accentuate health inequalities, and guided by ethical principles—Hong Kong as a case study. *International Medical Case Reports Journal, 1*(6), 1–9.

Woo, J. (2022a). Death among plenty—how disjointed policies failed older people living in residential care in times of COVID-19. *Journal of Medicine and Public Health, 3,* 1046.

Woo, J. (2022b). Healthcare for older people in Asia. *Age and Ageing, 51*(1). https://doi.org/10.1093/ageing/afab189

Woo, J. (2022c). Are COVID-19 Pandemic policies good for public health. *Medicine and Public Health 1*(1), 11–14. https://doi.org/10.56831/PSMPH-01-003

Woo, J., Chan, R., Leung, J., & Wong, M. (2010). Relative contributions of geographic, socioeconomic, and lifestyle factors to quality of life, frailty, and mortality in elderly. *PLoS One, 5*(1), e8775. https://doi.org/10.1371/journal.pone.0008775

Woo, J. & Chau, P. P. (2009). Aging in Hong Kong: The institutional population. *Journal of the American Medical Directors Association, 10*(7), 478–485. https://doi.org/10.1016/j.jamda.2009.01.009

Woo, J., Goggins, W., Sham, A., & Ho, S. C. (2005). Social determinants of frailty. *Gerontology, 51*(6), 402–408. https://doi.org/10.1159/000088705

Woo, J., Goggins, W., Zhang, X., Griffiths, S., & Wong, V. (2010). Aging and utilization of hospital services in Hong Kong: Retrospective cohort study. *International Journal of Public Health*, *55*(3), 201–207. https://doi.org/10.1007/s00038-009-0068-0

Woo, J., Leung, D., Yu, R., Lee, R., & Hung, W. (2021). Factors affecting trends in societal indicators of ageing well in Hong Kong: Policies, politics and pandemics. *The Journal of Nutrition, Health & Aging* 2021, *25*(3), 325–329. https://doi: 10.1007/s12603-020-1488-z

Woo, J., Lynn, H., Leung, J., & Wong, S. Y. (2008). Self-perceived social status and health in older Hong Kong Chinese women compared with men. *Women Health*, *48*(2), 209–234. https://doi.org/10.1080/03630240802313563

Woo, J., Yu, R., Cheung, K., & Lai, E. T. C. (2020). How much money is enough? Poverty and health in older people. *The Journal of Nutrition, Health & Aging*, *24*(10), 1111–1115.

Woo, J., Yu, R., Leung, G., Chiu, C., Hui, A., & Ho, F. (2021). An integrated model of community care for older adults: Design, feasibility and evaluation of impact and sustainability. *Aging Medicine and Healthcare*, *12*(3), 105–113. https://doi.org/10.33879/Amh.123.2021.07067

Woo, J., Yu, R., Wong, M., Yeung, Wong M., & Lum, C. (2015). Frailty screening in the community using the FRAIL Scale. *Journal of the American Medical Directors Association*, *16*(5), 412–419. https://doi.org/10.1016/j.jamda.2015.01.087

Woods, T., Palmarini, N., Corner, L., Barzilai, N., Bethell, L. J., Cox, L. S., Eyre, H., Ferrucci, L., Fried, L., Furman, D., Kennedy, B., Roddam, A., Scott, A., & Siow, R. C. (2022). Quantum healthy longevity for healthy people, planet, and growth. *The Lancet*

Healthy Longevity, *3*(12), e811–e813. https://doi.org/10.1016/S2666-7568(22)00267-7

World Health Organization. (2020). *Decade of healthy ageing: Baseline report*. Geneva: World Health Organization. https://www.who.int/publications/i/item/9789240017900

World Health Organization. (2021). *Global report on ageism*. Geneva: World Health Organization. http://www.who.int/publications/i/item/9789240016866

Yeoh, E. K. & Lai, H. Y. A. (2016). *An Investment for the Celebration of Aging*.

Yu, R., Leung, G., Leung, J., Cheng, C., Kong, S., Tam, L. Y., & Woo, J. (2022). Prevalence and distribution of intrinsic capacity and its associations with health outcomes in older people: The Jockey Club community eHealth care project in Hong Kong. *The Journal of Frailty & Aging*, *11*(3), 302–308. https://doi.org/10.14283/jfa.2022.19

Yu, R., Leung, G., & Woo, J. (2021). Randomized controlled trial on the effects of a combined intervention of computerized cognitive training preceded by physical exercise for improving frailty status and cognitive function in older adults. *International Journal of Environmental Research and Public Health*, *18*(4). https://doi.org/10.3390/ijerph18041396

Yu, R., Leung, J., Lum, C. M., Auyeung, T. W., Lee, J. S. W., Lee, R., & Woo, J. (2019). A comparison of health expectancies over 10 years: Implications for elderly service needs in Hong Kong. *International Journal of Public Health*, *64*(5), 731–742. https://doi.org/10.1007/s00038-019-01240-1

Yu, R., So, M. C., Tong, C., Ho, F., & Woo, J. (2020). Older adults' perspective towards participation in a multicomponent frailty prevention program: A qualitative study. *The Journal of Nutrition, Health & Aging, 24*(7), 758–764. https://doi.org/10.1007/s12603-020-1369-5

Yu, R., Tong, C., Ho, F., & Woo, J. (2020). Effects of a multicomponent frailty prevention program in prefrail community-dwelling older persons: A randomized controlled trial. *Journal of the American Medical Directors Association, 21*(2), 294.E291–294.E210. https://doi.org/10.1016/j.jamda.2019.08.024

Yu, R., Tong, C., Leung, J., & Woo, J. (2020). Socioeconomic inequalities in frailty in Hong Kong, China: A 14-year longitudinal cohort study. *International Journal of Environmental Research and Public Health, 17*(4). https://doi.org/10.3390/ijerph17041301

Yu, R., Cheung O, Leung J, et al. (2019). Is neighbourhood social cohesion associated with subjective well-being for older Chinese people? The neighbourhood social cohesion study. *BMJ Open, 9*(5), e023332. https://www.ncbi.nlm.nih.gov/pubmed/31079078